Total Health
& Weight Loss

The Truestar Way
Your guide to healthy living

Tim Mulcahy, CEO, Truestar Health
David Schleich, PhD, President, Truestar Health
Terry Nason, CFP, President, Truestar for Women
Michael Carrera, MSc
Joey Shulman, DC, RNCP
Natasha Turner, ND

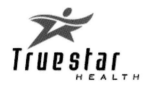

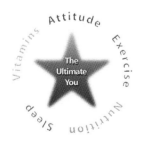

Vitamins · Attitude · Exercise · Nutrition · Sleep

The Ultimate You

Truestar Health Inc. and Quarry Press Inc.

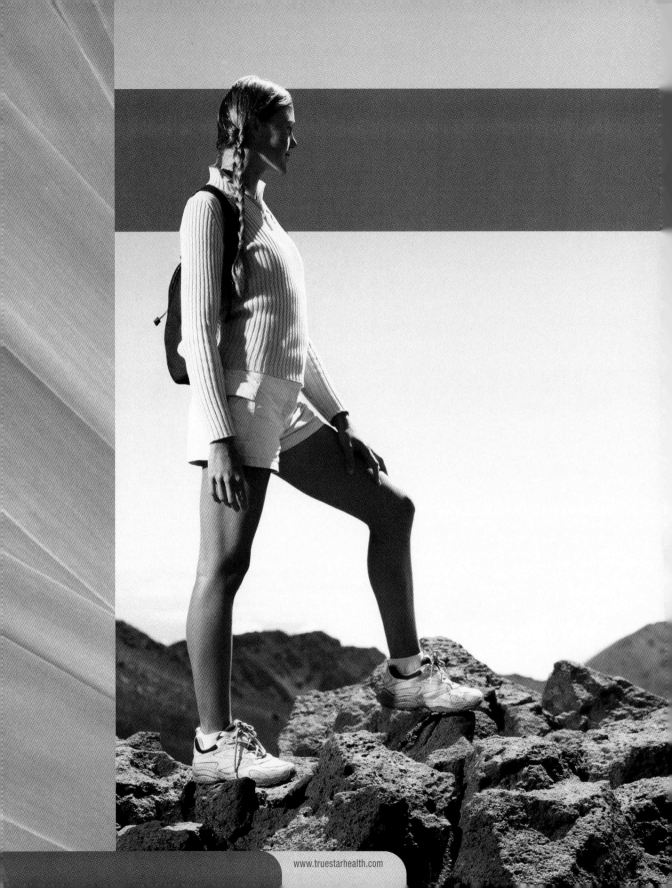

Welcome to
the Truestar Way …

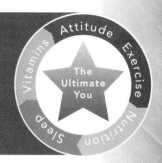

Truestar's total health and weight loss program is one of the most sophisticated systems outside of hiring your own naturopathic doctor and fitness trainer. And even if you were to do so, Truestar's proprietary weight loss supplements are only available through Truestarhealth.com or Truestar for Women Nutrition & Fitness Centers. The fact that we synergistically blend our nutrition, exercise, vitamin, attitude, and sleep programs is why we are the only company that pledges, "guaranteed weight loss or your money back."

A Lifestyle, not a Diet

The Truestar way is a *lifestyle*, not just a diet. Weight loss that is only diet-oriented can be effective, but never as effective as when you combine exercise and vitamins. Exercise alone is good, but weight loss will always be accelerated by adding in our supplements and a proper nutrition plan. For those who want to lose weight by only taking supplements, there is obviously some benefit, but faster and healthier results are achieved by adding in good nutrition and exercise. A positive attitude and techniques for empowering yourself by setting clear goals also make a difference, as does proper sleep to rejuvenate yourself each day. That's the Truestar way … good nutrition, exercise, supplements, attitude, and sleep … the five keys to healthy living blended synergistically.

Become the Ultimate You

By following the five points of this star, you can realize "The Ultimate You." We want you to become a Truestar all-star, like the many women of all ages who have joined our Truestar for Women Nutrition & Fitness Centers.

You will be amazed by their success stories. Not only have these women lost weight, they have gained confidence. They radiate health and vitality.

Here are some of the Truestar all-stars. Join them in following the Truestar way … Visit us soon at one of our centers, log on at www.truestarhealth.com, or call 1-888-448-TRUE

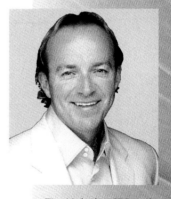

Tim Mulcahy, CEO and Founder of Truestar Health and Truestar for Women Nutrition & Fitness Centers

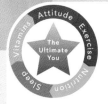

I feel great and look great, too!

How the Truestar Way Changed My Life

Like so many other women, I am a working mom who always puts her family and her job first. I raised three boys, and after each pregnancy, I kept the weight on instead of losing it. I made excuse after excuse, blaming my children or housework for not having enough time to look after myself. At one point, I tipped the scales at 230 pounds. I am 5 feet, 4 inches tall, and although I didn't look like I weighed 230 pounds (I tried to convince myself of this all the time), I hated looking at myself and refused to have my picture taken.

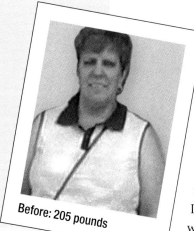

Before: 205 pounds

At one point, I tipped the scales at 230 pounds. I hated looking at myself and refused to have my picture taken.

I tried almost every diet on the market, which helped me to lose weight, but did nothing to keep it off. I followed the Diet Centre diet. I ate only salads and lost weight, but put the weight back on quickly when I stopped the diet. My next attempt to lose weight brought me to Weight Watchers. I followed the program and began to walk to work every day. I went down to 170 pounds. I was proud of myself and I was doing well until I experienced a series of family tragedies.

The first was the death of my mom from a brain aneurism. After her death, I was so worried about taking care of my father and the rest of my family that I stopped looking after myself. I put the

weight back on in no time. A few years later, my dad had a stroke. Taking care of him put even more responsibility on my shoulders, and I had absolutely no time for myself. Then, the worst thing that could happen to a parent happened to me. My youngest son, Daniel, died in a snowmobile accident. He was 18 at the time. I was devastated and felt like I had died too. For 2 years, I had a hard time caring about anything, let alone dieting and exercising.

Then last September, something changed in me. I decided that enough was enough and that I needed to get back my life and health. My blood pressure was high and so was my cholesterol level. I needed to do something about it. That's when I saw an advertisement for Truestar for Women Nutrition & Fitness Centers.

The Truestar program has all the right ingredients for a healthy lifestyle.
Thank you so much, Truestar, for giving me back my life!

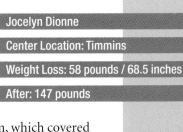

Jocelyn Dionne
Center Location: Timmins
Weight Loss: 58 pounds / 68.5 inches
After: 147 pounds

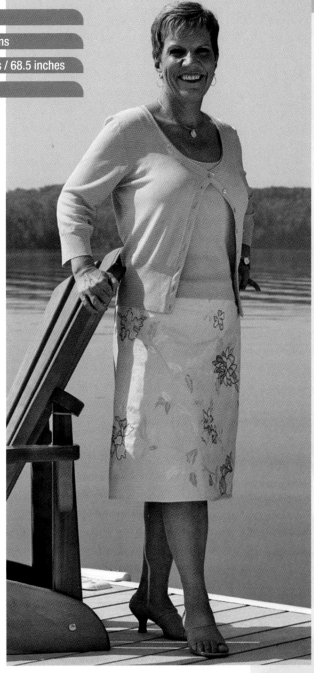

I thought their program, which covered nutrition, exercise, vitamins, attitude, and sleep, made sense. I decided to check them out. I was so impressed with their program that I signed up for a membership that same night.

I walked into Truestar last October weighing 205 pounds. Nine months later I reached my weight loss goal of 150 pounds. At my last weigh-in, I weighed 147 pounds and had lost 68.5 inches. I feel great and look great, too! My blood pressure and cholesterol levels are also back to normal.

I exercise five times a week and I am convinced that the weight will stay off for good. The Truestar program has all the right ingredients for a healthy lifestyle. They have nutrition plans, a fitness center, excellent supplements, and, most importantly, a coaching staff who have been there to support and guide me. They even have a program for sleeping better and keeping your attitude strong and positive. The staff have become like family to me. I look forward to seeing them every day.

Thank you so much, Truestar, for giving me back my life!

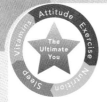

Where has Truestar been all my life?

How the Truestar Way Changed My Life

I am 60 years old and, wow, do I feel great! I have been at the Truestar for Women's Health & Fitness Center for 9 months and it has truly changed my life. I have learned to eat healthily and I am exercising. I also take the Truestar vitamins every day. Where has Truestar been all my life?

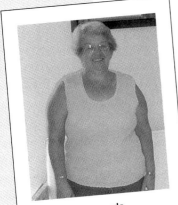

Before: 185 pounds

> When I look in the mirror, I just can't believe it's me!

Since joining this life-altering facility, I have lost 69 pounds and 78 inches. I am absolutely amazed at how much healthier and happier I feel. When I look in the mirror, I just can't believe it's me! I feel light and energetic. My husband loves the new me, but hates the new wardrobe expenses.

I have gone from a size 18 to a size 6. Shopping is now fun and exciting, not embarrassing.

Everyone has noticed the change in me. They all tell me that I look like a new person. I feel like a new person because I have changed my lifestyle, so, in turn, it has changed me as an individual. Never in my wildest dreams did I think people would call me "skinny." The last time someone called me skinny was in 1974! Needless to say, it has been a long time

since I have been at this weight. I have a full-time job at a Seniors Home. Everyone in the home thinks I am going to fade away, so they are keeping an eye on me.

My last visit to the doctor's office was exciting. Imagine that? My doctor told me that Truestar must be wonderful and successful because my medical condition was great inside and out.

The other day my husband and I went for a walk and ran into someone we had not seen in a while. She said hello to my husband, but didn't recognize me right away. When she finally clued in that it was me, she told my husband that she thought he was having an affair with a younger woman. I love it!

My family and friends are constantly giving me compliments. The personal coaches at Truestar are so proud of me and have been great role models to follow.

I am so pleased with my results. I never truly knew what it felt like to be healthy

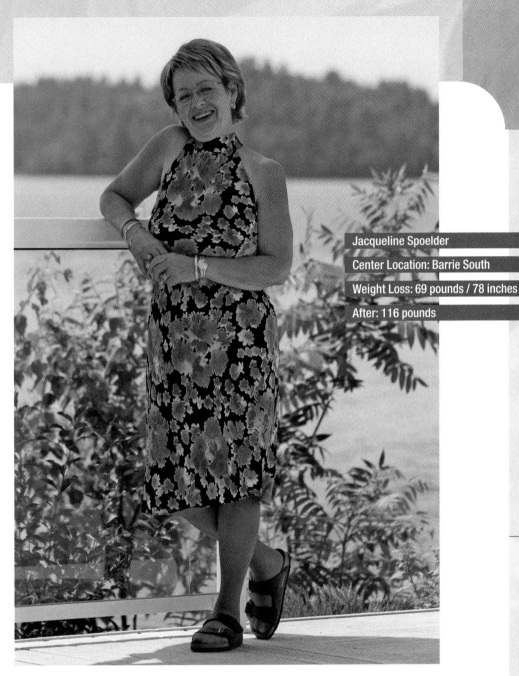

My birthday is on July 9th and I am looking forward to wearing a bikini for the first time in my life.

until now. I don't ever want to go back to feeling fat. This feeling of joy is so wonderful and overwhelming that I will never jeopardize it again.

My birthday is on July 9th and I am looking forward to wearing a bikini for the first time in my life.

I would like to thank Truestar for all the support and encouragement I needed to lose all this weight and to feel healthy.

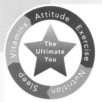

Your husband must love the new you!

How Truestar Way Changed My Life

What an amazing journey I have been on! It all began with my decision to join Truestar for Women. I knew I had to do something about my appearance and health because I wasn't happy. I was tired of yo-yo dieting.

After researching a number of diet programs, I was very impressed with Truestar's five key areas of healthy living — nutrition, exercise, vitamins, attitude, and sleep. Diabetes and cancer occur in my family. Truestar addressed these two illnesses directly. Believing in the program has made sticking to the program very easy.

Before joining Truestar, I allowed life's daily routines to interfere with my healthy living. I am a working mom and always felt guilty taking personal time for myself. I was pleasing everyone — but myself. Once I accepted the fact that I needed to take better care of myself, I started to look forward to the "me" time everyday. After my workouts, I would always leave in great spirits and with a clearer mind. I was

better prepared to meet my family's needs when I got home. Being fit and healthy make me a more energetic mom, wife, friend, and teacher.

The compliments I have received since losing 49 pounds are very flattering. My hard work and determination have all paid off. I keep receiving positive words of encouragement and praise. I am especially proud of the kind words my husband expresses to me because he has been my number one supporter during my weight-loss program. I vividly remember one night when we were cuddling and he remarked that he could feel my ribs. I was so thrilled. I also have to smile when people say to me, "Your husband must love the new you." I think he does!

> Before joining Truestar, I allowed life's daily routines to interfere with my healthy living.

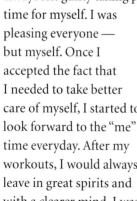

Before: 182 pounds

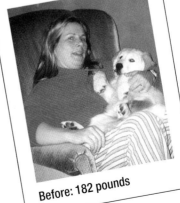

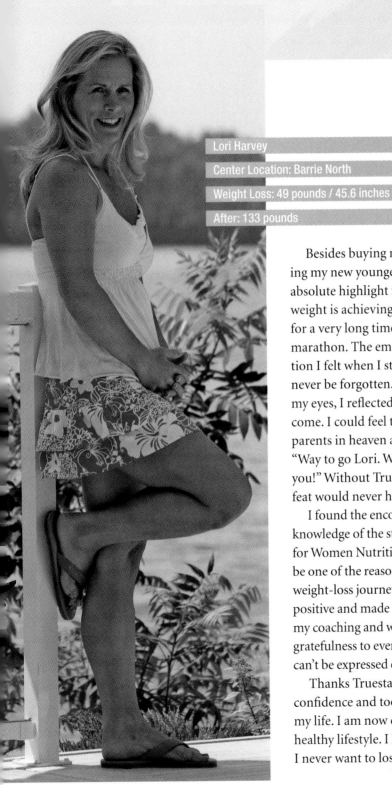

Lori Harvey

Center Location: Barrie North

Weight Loss: 49 pounds / 45.6 inches

After: 133 pounds

Besides buying new clothes and enjoying my new younger appearance, the absolute highlight for me of losing this weight is achieving a dream I had desired for a very long time — running a half marathon. The emotions and exhilaration I felt when I started my race will never be forgotten. As tears welled up in my eyes, I reflected upon how far I had come. I could feel the presence of my parents in heaven as they shouted, "Way to go Lori. We are so proud of you!" Without Truestar, this amazing feat would never have been realized.

I found the encouragement and knowledge of the staff at the local Truestar for Women Nutrition & Fitness Center to be one of the reasons for my successful weight-loss journey. Everyone was always positive and made me look forward to my coaching and workout sessions. My gratefulness to everyone who helped me can't be expressed enough.

Thanks Truestar for giving me the confidence and tools to take control of my life. I am now devoted to living a healthy lifestyle. I love the new me and I never want to lose this feeling!

The absolute highlight for me of losing this weight is achieving a dream I had desired for a very long time — running a half marathon.

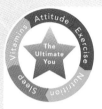

Contents

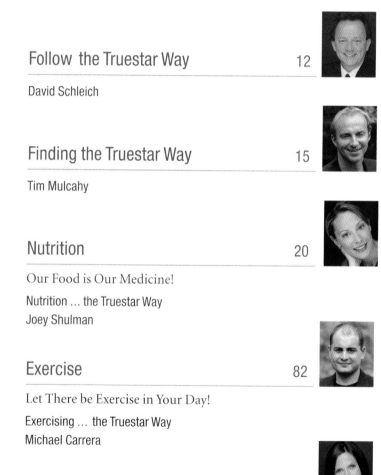
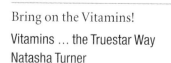

Foreword

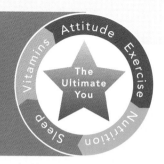

Follow the Truestar Way

Dr. David J. Schleich, PhD
President, Truestar Health Inc.
Former President, The Canadian College of Naturopathic Medicine

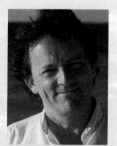

David J. Schleich

The daily experience of good health seems to be just out of reach for so many.

Obesity, late-onset diabetes, chronic fatigue, depression, and low energy levels are, unfortunately, commonplace in our communities, among our friends, our coworkers, and our families. Whether it is the high sugar content ketchup that accompanies the trans-fatty acid French fry one or two times a week, the habit of taking a convenient pill when a headache arrives, or getting caught in job pressures at the cost of balance and simplicity in our home lives, the daily experience of good health seems to be just out of reach for so many.

The State of Our Health

Our bodies build up the poisons, the stress, and the excess weight of our lifestyle choices. Those overloaded bodies and our spirit are all we have, in the end. The fanciest of cars, homes, wines, clothes, or flat-screen home theaters will not give us the most important wealth of all — a good state of health for mind and body.

Many North Americans squander their health over time, vaguely trusting that disease and pain will not arrive. We take our bodies for granted until something wakes us up to our vulnerabilities and then hope that the medical doctor can rectify the imbalance or the disease handily with drugs or surgery.

The truth is that despite the advances in medical science and the proliferation of weight loss and personal growth programs, many North Americans are not healthy. Our politicians and medical professionals tell us often that the health systems in North America are in trouble. They point to the high cost of health insurance in the United States, for example, or to the shortage of doctors and long waits in hospital emergency rooms in Canada. Governments and health insurers complain about constantly increasing drug costs.

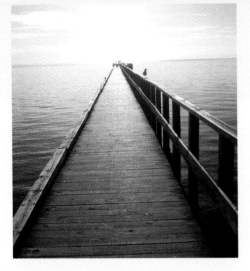

What can people do, then, to take care of their own health? The answer is to prevent health problems before they begin and to be vigilant about how lifestyle choices and environmental toxins threaten our well-being. And that's where Truestar Health comes in with reliable, enduring solutions to these problems.

Prevention

During my 7 years as the President of the Canadian College of Naturopathic Medicine, I saw over and over how *prevention* made all the difference. Naturopathic doctors teach their patients to prevent illness and disease by paying attention *every day* to the basic elements of healthy living: good nutrition, regular exercise, high-quality vitamins, good attitude, and healthy sleep habits. These five habits of highly healthy people are the foundation of the Truestar way to total health and weight loss.

Our mission at Truestar Health is to give people the keys to good health and lifelong well-being as inexpensively as possible. Truestar is dedicated to slicing through the confusing and conflicting health fads and trends that people glean from newspapers, television programs, and magazines. Truestar's objective is to provide sustained, professional guidance and true support for those wanting to change the quality of their lives forever.

The Truestar "way" is what our team of experts calls our approach to total health and weight loss. North Americans are accessing that "way" by the thousands through our company's remarkable website at www.truestarhealth.com, where over one million pages of health information are constantly refreshed, and through our rapidly expanding network of Truestar for Women Nutrition & Fitness Centers, where highly trained coaches work with members to plan a sustainable path to health and wellness. And now this book, *Total Health and Weight Loss the Truestar Way*. Our aim is to put solid, easy-to-understand information and tools in your hands right away.

North American baby boomers and their kids are better informed about the long-term dangers to health posed by lifestyle choices than any previous generation. They are seeking real ways to enter old age without the baggage of chronic disease and bodies that slow down prematurely or don't work at all. Many have found in the Truestar way a remarkable, integrated system built on sound knowledge and offered in simple, easy-to-follow guidelines. The Truestar way teaches people not to wait until disease or disability strikes. It teaches prevention; it teaches action.

Truestar's objective is to provide sustained, professional guidance and true support for those wanting to change the quality of their lives forever.

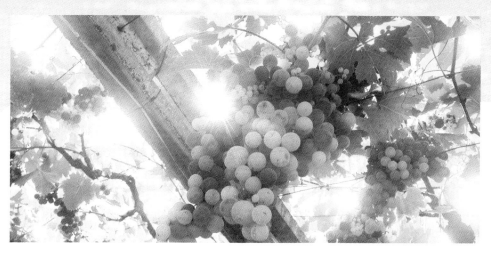

Lifelong Habits

What the Truestar way teaches is lifelong healthy habits for mind and body. The Truestar way is built on the conviction that the body, the spirit, and the mind have to work together throughout our lives. We are designed as living beings to know automatically and quickly about all kinds of changes inside and outside our bodies. Even though we sense right away when something hurts or doesn't work right, there are other developments in the body that are less obvious. They creep up on us gradually, such as when body fat accumulates, cholesterol sticks to our arteries, or chronic fatigue overcomes us at 4:00 in the afternoon. Meanwhile, our muscles get weak, our stomachs bloat with fat, our eyes need glasses, our ears need aids, and our feet need orthotic inserts at wildly high prices — and our bodies fail.

There is yet another bruise to our sense of well-being that affects so many — our anxiety about socially accepted images of what is beautiful, what is fashionably healthy, and what our bodies look like to others. We're never sure what the right path is or whether we have the discipline or self-love to follow it.

The Truestar way does not pull punches in providing guidance from here to there, from bodies in decline to bodies and spirits that are glowing with health. The Truestar way is as individual as we are. It's not just about losing 25 pounds or more. It's about learning to understand, respect, nourish, and fine-tune our bodies every day. Our coaches tell our members: "Learn and practice and believe and the weight loss will follow."

The Truestar way is built on the power of education. Backed by the most dynamic team of experts ever assembled in the disciplines of nutrition, exercise, vitamins, attitude, and sleep, the Truestar way can now become part of your life. When Tim Mulcahy, Truestar founder and fabulously successful Canadian entrepreneur, decided to share with people the elements of healthy living that are the foundation of his own achievements, he chose an integrated lifestyle approach. The Truestar way not only continues to fuel his own accomplishments, but also has energized thousands of people who have decided to change their lives forever. Try following the Truestar way for a while — we're sure you'll stay on this path for a lifetime.

Our coaches tell our members: "Learn and practice and believe and the weight loss will follow."

Try following the Truestar way for a while — we're sure you'll stay on this path for a lifetime.

Finding the Truestar Way

Tim Mulcahy
CEO and Founder of Truestar Health Inc.

One of the sobering joys of reaching mid-life is that we have the benefit of hindsight. We become more skilled and strategic about looking ahead, too. I have enormous gratitude for the success that has come my way in the past three decades. While I know that I created the momentum for some of that success, I also know that my mentors helped me to find my path. I've learned a lot from them and continue learning. What emerged as the Truestar way grew out of a commitment to lifelong learning that is stronger in me now than ever before.

Spiritual Success

By profession I am a direct sales entrepreneur. I have founded several highly successful companies over the years, including the Ontario Energy Savings Corp. (OESC), and trained thousands of sales agents. When a company is doing 240 sales meetings per year at the rate of five per week for 48 weeks, things can become monotonous. There are only so many closing techniques you can teach.

I found myself looking for something more than sales success. When I came across Dr Deepak Chopra's book, *The Seven Spiritual Laws of Success,* particularly his chapter on finding your purpose in life or your Dharma, I knew that I had found mine.

I envisioned a health service company whose mission would be to teach people to eat properly, exercise regularly, take high-quality vitamins, improve their attitude, and get a good night's sleep. I loved selling and felt that it was my Dharma to 'sell' good health.

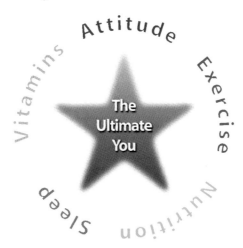

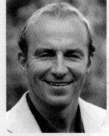

Tim Mulcahy

Five Principles of Good Health

The Truestar way began when I introduced my sales agents to good health practices as part of their job training and professional development. The name "Truestar" came from that original health program, based on the five keys to good health I envisioned, each key being the point of a 5-pointed star.

Nutrition, exercise, vitamins, attitude, sleep — combined, they represent the

> What emerged as the Truestar Way grew out of a commitment to lifelong learning that is stronger in me now than ever before.

Synergistic Personal Training System™ and the pathway to total health. My experience integrating these principles into my life has taught me that diligence in their use will generate benefits right away. Applying all five systematically to your life propels you to optimal health, wellness, and vitality. We may not be perfect in all five areas all of the time, but it is certainly an attainable goal with a large reward in personal empowerment and energy. When you become proficient in following the Truestar way, you become a True Star, which is something we are all born to be.

Dream Team

At Truestar, we have put together a dream team of health experts to help you find your own path to total health and weight loss. I was determined to recruit the best possible health team. We needed a top-notch naturopathic doctor to head up our Vitamin and Sleep divisions, an exceptional exercise science expert for our Exercise division, and an accomplished nutritionist for our Nutrition division. Ably assisted by Alison Greiner, I would oversee the Attitude section largely because I had been training people in that area for many years. We also needed an inspirational business-woman and fitness expert to head up our Truestar for Women Nutrition & Fitness Center division. Our search was successful.

Dr Natasha Turner (ND) is a graduate of The Canadian College of Naturopathic Medicine, one of the continent's leading complementary and alternative medicine schools. Before coming to Truestar, she had a thriving private practice and had also been doing innovative consulting work with the Sports Clubs of Canada. She contributes two chapters to this book — *Vitamins … the Truestar Way* and *Sleep… the Truestar Way.*

Dr Tudor Bompa (PhD) has been called a 'god' in the fitness industry. The author of *Periodization,* a guide to phased-based training, Dr Bompa has set up training systems for the Australian Olympic Team, the Argentine soccer team, the St. Louis Blues hockey team, and Lennox Lewis, the former world champion heavyweight boxer. We retained Dr Bompa as a senior consultant, and he recommended Michael Carrera (MSc) as one of the brightest minds in the fitness industry to head up our Exercise section. Michael and Tudor have developed one the most extensive online exercise programs in the world with help from 'teammates' Reggie Reyes and Natasha Vani. Michael contributes a chapter on *Exercise … the Truestar Way.*

Dr Joey Shulman (DC, RNCP) is the author of *Winning the Food Fight: Every Parent's Guide to Raising a Healthy, Happy Child.* Joey became our VP of Nutrition, and we quickly added two

---

Nutrition, exercise, vitamins, attitude, sleep — combined, they represent the Synergistic Personal Training System™ and the pathway to total health.

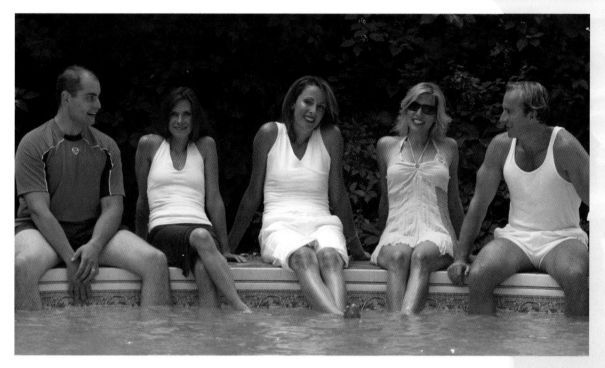

nutritionists to her team, Alana Gold and Sofia Segounis. Joey contributes a chapter on *Nutrition … the Truestar Way*.

I first met Terry Nason (CFP) at a hockey tournament, where our daughters were playing. A certified financial planner, she so impressed me with her enthusiasm for womens' health and fitness that we hired her as president of our health and fitness centers. Terry contributes a chapter on *Women's Health & Fitness … the Truestar Way*. She is also the woman you see working out in the Exercise chapter — and the model of good health and vitality you see on the cover of the book.

The Truestar Website

We were off and running. Our goal was to provide the most extensive information on nutrition, exercise, vitamins, attitude, and sleep available anywhere. We accomplished just that.

With a great sense of creativity and commitment supported by many hours of plain old hard work from our health and IT teams, we built the world's most comprehensive healthy lifestyle website. Although the main focus of our current growth is our nutrition and fitness centers, the Truestar website remains the foundation, the backbone, the framework of our program. I have yet to see anything comparable.

At Truestar, we have put together a dream team of health experts to help you find your own path to total health and weight loss.

Truestar Health is unique in providing a cutting edge personal profiling system that takes into consideration your age, sex, height, weight, activity level, medical history, and health or weight-loss goals and provides a personal plan just for you.

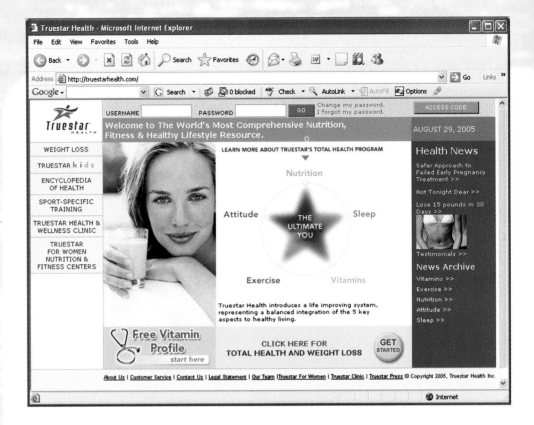

Nutrition

☐ BALANCED MEAL PLANS

Over 10,000 calorically, hormonally, and pH balanced meal plans for all ages and dietary requirements, including homemade meals and "on the go" meals

☐ WEIGHT-LOSS TRACKING CHART

A personal weight-loss tracking chart for recording weight and inches lost

☐ FOODTRAKKER

A personal program that breaks down the nutritional content of over 100,000 foods and meal combinations

☐ CUSTOMIZED SHOPPING LIST

A printable shopping list based upon members' meal plans

☐ GLYCEMIC INDEX AND GLYCEMIC LOAD CHARTS

An extensive list of common foods to use in selecting healthy carbohydrates

Exercise

☐ EXERCISE VIDEOS

More than 3000 exercise videos, for ages 6 to 86

☐ WORKOUT REGIMES

More than 15,000 workouts for beginners, intermediates, and pros

☐ SPORTS TRAINING PROGRAMS

Specific training programs for 20 of the world's most popular sports, again for all ages

☐ TV WATCHING WORKOUT

20-minute workouts, including the popular "TV watching workout"

Vitamins

☐ VITAMIN PROFILE

A full personal vitamin profiling system that helps you to choose the right vitamin for your type of body and lifestyle

☐ VITAMIN GUIDE

A program for selecting professional series vitamins and supplements for weight loss and good health, with videos explaining the benefits of each

☐ DRUG INTERACTION CHART

A guide to the safety and risks, as well as the interactions and contraindications, in using drugs and vitamins

Attitude

☐ DAILY LIFE IMPROVEMENT CHECKLIST

A guide to setting out on a new way of life, including a sophisticated nutrition scoring system

☐ PERSONAL GOAL SETTING PROGRAM

A customized guide to establishing realistic goals and achieving them successfully

☐ INSPIRATIONAL QUOTATIONS AND APHORISMS

A saying a day to keep your goals focused and your spirits high

Sleep

☐ MOTIVATIONAL CHILDREN'S BEDTIME STORIES

I personally listen to them — they're good!

☐ MEDITATION CDS

You can meditate on being on a beach, on Mars, or in prehistoric time

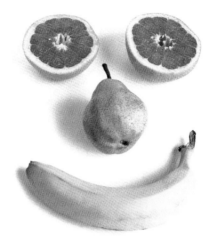

☐ SLEEP TIPS

Quick and easy hints and plans for getting a good night's sleep

Bonuses

☐ An Encyclopedia of Health
☐ Daily health newsletters
☐ Thousands of articles relating to the most relevant health issues
☐ … and much, much, much more

We launched the website in September 2003. We now have members from all around the world — we've had people sign up from Saudi Arabia, Kazakhstan, the Far East, and Scandinavia, with the largest contingent from the United States and Canada.

This book condenses the 1.2 million pages of information available at truestarhealth.com into just over 200 pages — a tight but convenient fit. Once you've read this book — or even as you read along — you will be tempted to visit the website for more information. We'll be waiting there, ready to help you.

The Truestar website remains the foundation, the backbone, the framework of our program. I have yet to see anything comparable.

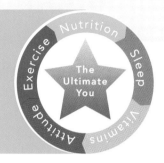

Our Food Is Our Medicine!

Tim Mulcahy

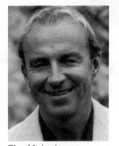

Tim Mulcahy

I was at the top of
my game. This can't
be happening to me,
I thought, so I began
to look for answers.

Some time ago, I was driving to a sales meeting when I experienced what I thought was a heart attack. I pulled over, caught my breath, and then I drove to the hospital, where they calmed me down and told me it was only an anxiety attack. I was 25 at the time, enjoying business success as the owner of Toronto Water Filters. I was at the top of my game. This can't be happening to me, I thought, so I began to look for answers.

One of my employees suggested I see a naturopathic doctor by the name of James D'Adamo, whose son has since gained some fame for his *Eat Right 4 Your Type* diet. After Dr D'Adamo took my blood and looked at a strand of my hair, he told me I was borderline hypoglycemic and very sensitive to insulin. This could lead to adult onset diabetes and heart disease. He suggested I cut out pizza, pasta, and beer from my diet and instead go on a fairly strict protein diet. He also advised me to exercise every morning. Well, I tried to stick to the diet, but didn't have the discipline. I loved Italian food and beer too much.

A few years later, I began to feel tired all of the time after I ate. I hated losing the energy I needed for my business, and began reading more books on diet to see if I could solve this problem. Some books said that if I ate pasta, I would gain energy. Other books said that I should only eat fruit until noon. I was struggling with mixed messages. One day, I picked up *The Zone Diet* audio CD by Dr Barry Sears and listened to it on my commute from the office. The information made sense to me immediately. Dr Sears really hit home when he said, "If you eat and feel good afterwards, without losing energy, you ate right; whereas if you eat and feel tired afterwards, you didn't eat right."

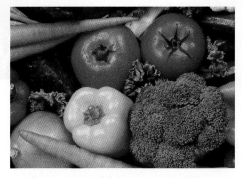

The theory behind *The Zone* is maintaining hormonal balance in the body, which means that each meal should combine fairly equal amounts of healthy carbohydrates, lean protein, and 'good' fat found in such foods as olive oil, almonds, and avocados. Most meals are too high in starchy carbohydrates that are quickly converted to sugar (glucose) in your blood and make your insulin levels spike. This results in feeling tired and possible weight gain. Overeating has the same effect, which explained for me why at Thanksgiving and other celebrations when we eat way too much, we want to go to sleep soon afterwards.

That was not far off from what Dr D'Adamo had recommended almost a decade earlier. But now, I was more receptive to the information. I was tired of being tired after eating. I knew there was a better way.

I've eaten in this manner ever since, with the odd exception from time to time — Italian food is so seductive! I've also fed my family this way and educated them on the pitfalls of diets too high in carbohydrates, including sodas and sugary drinks. I recall eating Fruit Loops or Alpha Bits for breakfast as a child and going to school and wanting to have a nap right there at the desk. Maintaining a high energy level is beneficial in all situations — learning, working, parenting, socializing, exercising, or relaxing. The first piece of the health puzzle was now in place for me. Eating right became a fundamental part of the Truestar way to lifelong health and wellness.

Eating right became a fundamental part of the Truestar way to lifelong health and wellness.

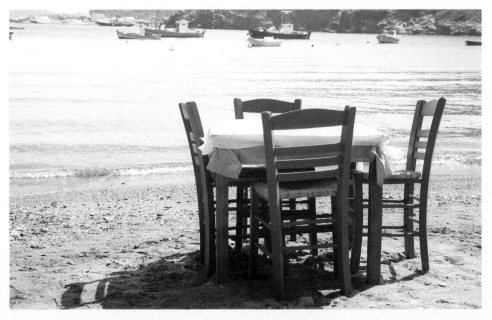

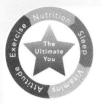

Nutrition . . . the Truestar Way

Dr Joey Shulman
DC, Registered Nutritionist, Vice-President, Nutrition

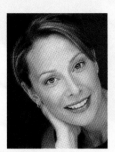

Joey Shulman

The quality and quantity of the food we eat has a direct impact on our health. Depending on our food choices, nutrition can be the underlying cause of various sicknesses and diseases or, alternatively, can be the springboard to a life filled with health, wellness, and vigor.

Nutrition is the fundamental component of the Truestar five-fold approach to the elements of good health — nutrition, exercise, vitamins, attitude, and sleep. Unfortunately, our personal health is being challenged and our health-care system is undergoing enormous strain because of the rise in the consumption of processed 'fake' foods, such as trans fatty acids, refined flours, and fast food. No longer are we witnessing nutritional deficiency diseases, such as rickets (a lack of vitamin D) or scurvy (a lack of vitamin C). Instead, the prevalent disease processes of the 21st century are 'gluttony diseases'. Due to eating too much of the wrong types of foods, we are seeing a rise in the prevalence of many common diseases and health conditions.

DIET-RELATED DISEASES

- Obesity (adult and child)
- Type II Diabetes (adult onset and child onset)
- Cancer
- Heart disease
- Stroke
- Atherosclerosis
- Asthma
- Allergies
- Depression

Information Is Power

Our mission at Truestar is to provide you with the 'need-to-know' information for establishing good nutrition and permanent weight loss. The pleasant side effect of eating right can be the prevention or reversal of disease processes. This nutritional knowledge is easy to apply to your day-to-day eating habits, allowing you to

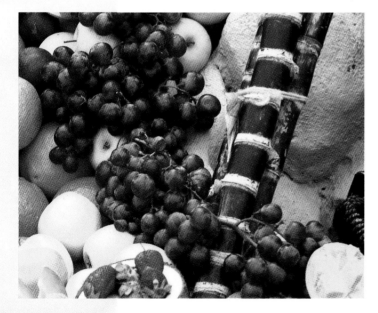

achieve a lean and fit body, high energy levels, and overall vitality. Whether your goal is to lose weight, build muscle, or protect against various illnesses, our programs have been designed to shift you easily into this new nutritional lifestyle.

We'll begin with some 'big' ideas about carbohydrates, protein, and fats — the three macronutrients necessary in every diet. Don't be intimidated by these ideas; we'll make them easy to understand and, even more importantly, easy to apply to your diet. Then we'll present the Truestar diet program, a three-phase approach to weight loss that is personal, adaptive, and proven to work. Truestar's

eating for success guidelines and delicious recipes will provide the final leg to complete this stage of your health journey. Are you ready? Let's begin!

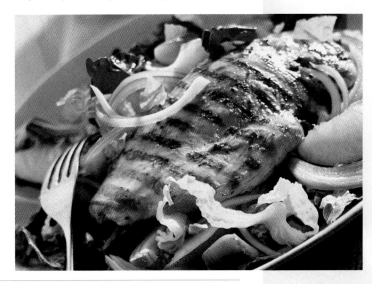

The Group of 3

Carbohydrates, Proteins, & Fats

Let's start with the 'macro' and 'micro' basics. Food is composed of three macronutrients — namely, carbohydrates, proteins, and fats — and a host of micronutrients — chiefly, vitamins and minerals. A relatively large amount of each of these three macronutrients is required daily in order for the body to run smoothly. Micronutrients are needed in smaller amounts in the diet, but are also crucial in achieving optimal health. Here, we will focus on macronutrients, and in the Bring on the Vitamins! chapter, my colleague, Dr Natasha Turner, will provide you with what you need to know about micronutrients.

When it comes to nutrition, knowledge is power. A basic understanding of how macronutrients work in the body and how to obtain them in the diet is a key factor in your path to achieving your optimal weight. The Truestar nutritional philosophy is based on the proper combination of all three macronutrients. No one macronutrient is 'demonized'. Not all fats are bad, for example. Indeed, some are essential. The Truestar program is not an anti-carbohydrate or a pro-protein diet. No one macronutrient is excluded at the expense of another. But some forms of macronutrients are better than others.

Whether your goal is to lose weight, build muscle, or protect against various illnesses, our programs have been designed to shift you easily into this new nutritional lifestyle.

FOOD BALANCE

In order to achieve your ideal body weight, feel energetic, and ward off illness, your meals and snacks should break down into the following proportions of carbohydrates, proteins, and fats.

☐ 40% low glycemic index carbohydrates
☐ 30% lean proteins
☐ 30% essential fats

What do we mean by 'low glycemic index' carbohydrates, 'lean' protein, and 'essential fatty acids'? Read on!

Carbohydrates

Carbohydrates are found in plants and plant products — fruits, vegetables, legumes, and grains, such as oatmeal, rice, cereal, bread, and pasta.

Carbohydrates are broken down in the body into glucose (blood sugar) and are utilized as the primary source of fuel. The glucose derived from carbohydrates is then transferred into the cells and used for energy. In fact, certain parts of the body, such as the brain or red blood cells, rely exclusively on glucose from carbohydrates as their only energy source. Other parts of the body can use others sources of fuel, such as fat or protein, but none burn as efficiently and cleanly as carbohydrates.

Recently, carbohydrates have received some undeserved bad press due to the popularity of high-protein diets, such as the Atkins and the South Beach programs. In reality, carbohydrates are critical in sustaining our energy and vitality throughout the day. Without them, our health would suffer.

Good Carbs, Bad Carbs

Many people are eating too much of the wrong type of carbohydrates, such as refined flours and sugars, without even realizing the detrimental effects they have on health. White bread, pasta, rice, cereal, cookies, muffins, ice cream, and soda pop are just a few of the culprits showing up on our grocery store shelves and ending up in our daily diet.

With food manufacturers cleverly disguising products that contain an abundant amount of white sugar and white flour, these processed foods are very difficult to avoid, unless you are an informed consumer. The key to eating carbohydrates without gaining weight and having them affect mood, cravings, or energy levels does not involve eliminating them completely, rather in deciphering the good type from the bad.

Even when we are able to distinguish the 'bad' from the 'good' carbohydrates, many people are throwing up their

Log on to www.truestarhealth.com to create a personal nutritional meal plan based on your weight-loss goals, physical activity level, and current health status.

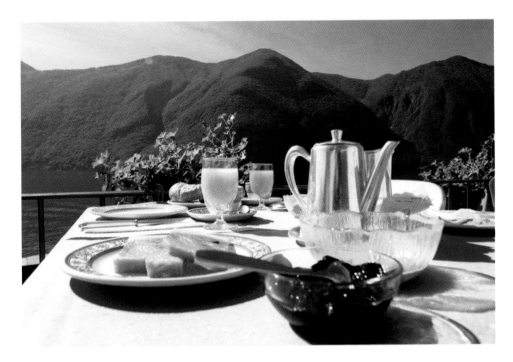

hands in nutritional bewilderment about how much carbohydrates they should eat each day. Who can blame them? Even the established food guidelines (Canada's Food Guide to Healthy Eating from Health Canada and the USDA Food Guide Pyramid Guide to Daily Food Choices) offer contradictory and outdated recommendations. The 6-11 servings of bread, cereal, rice, and pasta recommended are far too much! Let's have a further look at the world of carbohydrates.

Slow Down the Insulin!

Eating carbohydrates properly lies in understanding the intricate relationship between blood sugar (glucose) levels and insulin. Insulin is a hormone secreted from the pancreas in response to elevated blood glucose levels. One of insulin's many roles in the body is to transport glucose into the cells. The process works in the following manner:

Blood glucose levels are elevated by eating a specific food

▼

The pancreas responds by secreting insulin

▼

Insulin opens up the gates of cells to allow glucose to be absorbed and used for energy

▼

Glucose gets absorbed into the cells

▼

Blood glucose levels are normalized

If you have ever experienced a falling of energy 1 to 3 hours following a meal, you are likely in a state of hypoglycemia, which includes symptoms of fatigue, moodiness, hunger, mental fogginess, and, ironically, cravings for more carbohydrates.

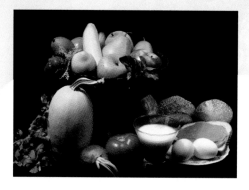

Glycemic Index

Categories

Low (up to 55)

Medium (56 to 70)

High (over 70)

So why all the fuss about carbohydrates, weight gain, and low carb foods? It is because certain foods, such as refined flours and sugars, cause an over-secretion of insulin. When insulin is over-secreted, a 'crash' in blood sugar levels occurs, sending the poor individual who has just eaten them into a state of hypoglycemia (low blood sugar).

If you have ever experienced a falling of energy 1 to 3 hours following a meal, you are likely in a state of hypoglycemia, which includes symptoms of fatigue, moodiness, hunger, mental fogginess, and, ironically, cravings for more carbohydrates. To top it all off and make matters worse, excess glucose is stored as fat, resulting in weight gain. To prevent these problems, we need to eat carbohydrates that do not cause an over-secretion of insulin.

Low Glycemic Index Carbs

To avoid weight gain and energy fluctuations, it is best to eat carbohydrates that are rated low on a scale called the glycemic index. The glycemic index measures the speed of entry of glucose (sugar) from a carbohydrate into the bloodstream. The faster the speed of entry, the more insulin the body will secrete in response.

For ranking purposes, the glycemic index is divided into three categories: low, medium, and high. Food is categorized on a scale of 0 to 100, depending on its effect on blood sugar levels. On the glycemic scale, the highest measurement is for glucose, which has the ranking of 100. For the most part, foods that are lowest on the glycemic index have the slowest rate of entry into the bloodstream, and therefore have the lowest insulin response.

Processed foods, such as white flour products, certain fruits, candies, and

SUGAR CONTENT OF COMMON FOODS

Food	Teaspoons of Sugar	% Daily Value
Snickers bar (2.1 oz or 59 g)	5 3/4	58%
Low-fat, fruit-flavored yogurt (8 oz or 226 g)	7	70%
Pepsi (12 oz or 340 ml)	10 1/4	103%
Pancake syrup (1/4 cup or 59 ml)	10 1/4	103%
Hostess lemon fruit pie (4 1/2 oz or 127 g)	11 1/4	115%
McDonald's vanilla shake (20 oz or 568 ml)	12	120%
Cinnabon (7 1/4 oz or 205 g)	12 1/4	123%
Strawberry Fruitopia (20 oz or 568 ml)	17 3/4	178%
Dairy Queen, Mr. Misty Slush (32 oz or 909 ml)	28	280%

(Information provided by Centre for Science in the Public Interest, August 1999)

cakes, tend to have a higher glycemic index rating. For example:

- ☐ Plain white baguette   95
- ☐ Strawberry cupcake   73
- ☐ White bread   73
- ☐ White bagel   72

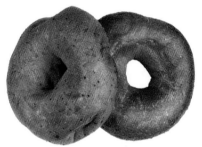

Protein, fat, and especially the fiber found primarily in unprocessed carbohydrates act as brakes to slow the entry of glucose from a particular food into the bloodstream. Most fresh vegetables, beans, and whole grains are full of fiber, which is reflected by a lower glycemic index rating. For example:

- ☐ Green peas   48
- ☐ Boiled black-eyed peas   42
- ☐ All bran   38

The glycemic index is a tool and not necessarily reflective of healthy foods for all categories. For example, M & M's have a low glycemic index rating due to their high fat content.

Glycemic Load

Because the glycemic index can reflect occasional inaccuracies in terms of insulin response, the glycemic load is perhaps more useful in choosing healthy carbohydrates for your diet. The glycemic load considers a food's glycemic index and the amount of carbohydrates per serving.

GLYCEMIC INDEX AND LOAD		
Value	Glycemic Index	Glycemic Load
High:	70 or more	20
Medium:	56-69	11-19
Low:	55 or less	10 or less

Glycemic Load Calculation

The glycemic load (GL) is the glycemic index (GI) divided by 100 and multiplied by its available carbohydrate content.

CARROTS

Let's take the example of carrots — a highly nutritional food choice. While carrots have received some undeserved bad press due to their high glycemic index rating of 71, a typical serving of one carrot has only has 4 grams of carbohydrates.

71 GI x 0.04 grams = 2.84 GL

Therefore, carrots have a low glycemic load rating.

WHITE PASTA

Now let's take the example of 1 cup of cooked, white pasta that also has a glycemic index rating of 71, but contains 40 grams of carbohydrates, 10 times more than the serving of carrots.

71GI x 0.40 grams = 28.7 GL

Therefore, pasta has a high glycemic load because it is carbohydrate-dense.

BEWARE

A majority of whole wheat bread or pasta is a refined flour item that simply has had black strap molasses added to make it appear brown. Tricky marketing, isn't it? These food items have a higher glycemic index rating and can lead to a state of hypoglycemia and weight gain. When purchasing grain items, such as bread, check the label to ensure the product has been made with 100% whole-grain flour. As a crude test, the bread should actually feel slightly heavier and needs to be chewed in your mouth a little more to break down the fiber.

Glycemic Index and Glycemic Load

Fruits & Fruit Product

Food item	Glycemic Index (GI)	Serving size (g)	Glycemic Load (GL)
Apples, raw	34	120	5
Apricots	57	120	5
Banana, ripe	51	120	13
Banana, under-ripe	30	120	6
Banana, over-ripe	48	120	12
Cherries	22	120	3
Cranberry juice	68	250	24
Dates, dried	103	60	42
Figs, dried	61	60	16
Grapefruit	25	120	3
Grapefruit juice unsweetened	48	250	9
Grapes	46	120	8
Grapes, black	59	120	11
Kiwi fruit	53	120	6
Lychee, canned in syrup	79	120	16
Mango	51	120	8
Marmalade orange	48	30	9
Oranges	42	120	5
Orange juice	52	250	12
Papaya	59	120	10
Peach	42	120	5
Peach, in heavy syrup	58	120	9
Pear	38	120	4
Pear halves, in syrup	25	120	4
Pineapple	59	120	7
Plum	39	120	5
Prunes, pitted	29	60	10
Raisins	64	60	28
Cantaloupe	65	120	4
Strawberries, fresh	40	120	1
Strawberry jam	51	30	10
Sultanas	56	60	25
Tomato juice, no sugar added	38	250	4
Watermelon	72	120	4

Glycemic Index and Glycemic Load

Vegetables

Food item	Glycemic Index (GI)	Serving size (g)	Glycemic Load (GL)
Broad beans	79	80	9
Green peas	48	80	3
Pumpkin	75	80	3
Sweet corn	54	80	9
Beet root	64	80	5
Carrots	71	80	3
Cassava, boiled	46	100	12
Parsnips	97	80	12
Baked potato	85	150	26
White potato, cooked	50	150	14
French fries, frozen	75	150	22
Instant mashed potato	85	150	17
New potato	57	150	12
Sweet potato	61	150	17

Legumes and Nuts

Food item	Glycemic Index (GI)	Serving size (g)	Glycemic Load (GL)
Black-eye beans, boiled	42	150	13
Chick peas, boiled	28	150	8
Navy beans	38	150	12
Kidney beans, boiled	28	150	7
Black beans, cooked	20	150	5
Lentil, green, boiled	30	150	5
Lentil, red, dried	26	150	5
Lima beans, frozen	32	150	10
Mung bean, cooked	42	150	7
Peas, dried, boiled	22	150	2
Pinto beans, dried	39	150	10
Romano beans	46	150	8
Soya beans, boiled	15	150	1
Split peas, boiled	32	150	6

Glycemic Index and Glycemic Load

Breads

Food item	Glycemic Index (GI)	Serving size (g)	Glycemic Load (GL)
Bagel, white frozen	72	70	25
Baguette, white, plain	95	30	15
French baguette with chocolate spread	72	70	27
French baguette with butter and strawberry jam	62	70	26
Coarse barley kernel bread	27	30	5
Buckwheat bread	47	30	10
Hamburger bun	61	30	9
Kaiser roll	73	30	12
Gluten free multi-grain bread	79	30	10
Pumpernickel bread	46	30	5
Light rye	68	30	10
White spelt wheat bread	74	30	17
Spelt multi-grain bread	54	30	7
White flour	70	30	10
100% whole grain bread	51	30	7

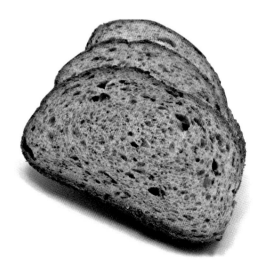
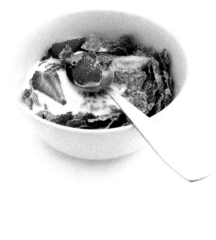

Glycemic Index and Glycemic Load

Breakfast Cereals

Food item	Glycemic Index (GI)	Serving size (g)	Glycemic Load (GL)
All Bran ™	30	30	4
Bran Chex ™	58	30	11
Cheerios ™	74	30	15
Corn Bran ™	75	30	15
Cornflakes ™ (Kellogg's)	92	30	24
Corn Pops ™ (Kellogg's)	80	31	21
Cream of Wheat ™ (Nabisco)	66	250	17
Crispix ™ (Kellogg's)	87	30	22
Froot Loops ™ (Kellogg's)	69	30	18
Frosted Flakes ™ (Kellogg's)	55	30	15
Grapenuts ™ (Kraft)	67	30	13
Just Right ™ (Kellogg's)	60	30	13
Mini Wheats ™ (Kellogg's)	72	30	15
Muesli, (No Name)	60	30	11
Oat bran, raw	59	10	3
Porridge	69	250	16
Rice Krispies ™ (Kellogg's)	82	30	21

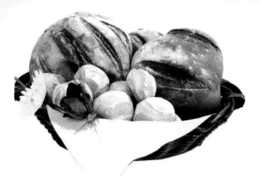

Low GI vs High GI Foods

To understand how the glycemic index of foods affects blood sugar, let's consider the following two examples.

HIGH GI DIET

Person A eats a chocolate chip muffin and coffee for lunch in order to curb her hunger and cravings. Due to the high sugar content and processing of the flour in the muffin, the sugar enters the blood stream at a rushing speed. The muffin and coffee have a high glycemic index and load rating, which causes glucose (sugar) to zoom into the bloodstream. In response to this situation, the pancreas secretes insulin to deal with the large amount of sugar.

Now, if this situation occurs once or twice, an appropriate amount of insulin is secreted. However, if your diet is filled with processed flours and sugars, the pancreas becomes de-sensitized and will secrete more and more insulin to deal with the excess sugar. Excess insulin will result in hypo-glycemic (low blood sugar) symptoms, such as fatigue, mood swings, and brain 'fog', as well as leading to weight gain and even the development of type II diabetes.

LOW GI DIET

Now, let us consider a second scenario. Person B eats a perfectly balanced meal consisting of low glycemic carbohydrates, lean proteins, and essential fats. She eats a tuna sandwich on whole grain bread with half a handful of almonds for lunch. Because this meal is perfectly balanced, the blood sugar (glucose) trickles, not rushes, into the blood stream. In response, an appropriate amount of insulin is released.

The result? Energy is maintained, weight is not gained, and Person B goes on with her day feeling focused and alert. See the difference?

Sample Serving Sizes

Depending on activity level, the average amount of carbohydrates that should be consumed daily for adult men and women ranges from 80 to 100 grams per day for women and 100 to 150 grams for men.

What do serving sizes look like?

- A palm (without fingers or thumb) or a deck of cards = 3-ounce serving of meat
- A thumb tip = 1 teaspoon
- Three thumb tips = 1 tablespoon
- One thumb = 25 g of most cheeses (A typical serving is approximately two thumbs)
- A fist = 1 cup

Recommended Servings

FRUIT
- 1 serving of fruit = $1/2$ cup or 1 small fruit = 10 grams of carbohydrates

VEGETABLES
- 1 serving of vegetables = 1 cup = 5 grams of carbohydrates

BEANS
- 1 serving of beans = $1/2$ cup = 20-25 grams of carbohydrates

WHOLE GRAINS
- 1 serving of whole grains = 1 whole-wheat tortilla = 12 grams of carbohydrates
- 1 serving of whole grains = 2 pieces of crisp Wasa bread = 15 grams of carbohydrates
- 1 serving of whole grains = 1 slice of whole-wheat bread = 15 grams of carbohydrates
- 1 serving of whole grains = 1 whole-wheat bagel = 25-40 grams of carbohydrates depending on density

The Truestar Way to Eat Carbohydrates

EAT:
- Low glycemic-index fruits, such as raspberries, blueberries, strawberries, melon, papaya, and cherries.
- Low glycemic-index and nutrient-rich vegetables, such as broccoli, cauliflower, celery, cucumbers, tomatoes, spinach, peppers, eggplant, sweet potatoes, squash, and zucchini.
- Low glycemic-index and high-fiber content beans, such as kidney beans, black beans, navy beans, and chick peas
- Whole grains, such as oatmeal, kamut, or spelt pasta bread, and brown rice, in moderation.

DON'T EAT:
- Refined and processed grains, such as white bread, pasta, rice, and potatoes (mashed or baked white potato), because these products are rated high on the glycemic index and will promote weight gain and fluctuations in blood sugar levels
- Refined sugary foods, such as cakes, cookies, muffins, soda pop, and candy

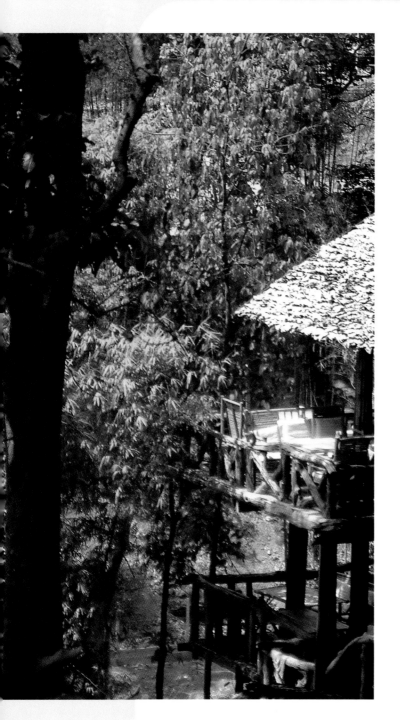

Proteins

Proteins are the second category of macronutrients that are a necessary part of every diet. The building blocks of proteins are called amino acids. There are 22 amino acids in total. Thirteen are *non-essential*, meaning the body can synthesize them and they do not have to be derived from food sources. Nine are classified as *essential*, meaning the body cannot synthesize them, so they must come from our diet.

Proteins serve many functions in the body, such as maintaining proper growth and repair of muscles and tissues; manufacturing hormones, antibodies, and enzymes; and preserving the proper pH (acid-alkaline) balance in the body.

Weight Loss

In terms of weight loss, proteins have the opposite effect of carbohydrates. When eating a protein, the hormone glucagon is secreted. Unlike excess insulin that is stored as fat, glucagon facilitates the breakdown of fat. Although both insulin and glucagon are necessary hormonal reactions that occur from eating specific foods, when either one is secreted in excess, health suffers.

Sample Serving Sizes of Protein

As a general rule, the amount of protein that should be consumed daily for adult men and women ranges from 80 to 120 grams per day (20 to 25 grams for women per meal and 30 to 35 grams for men per meal). If you are weight training, your protein requirements increase.

Recommended Servings

To measure protein servings, use this rule of 'thumb': the palm of your hand without thumb or fingers or a deck of cards = 3 ounces of protein

- ☐ 1 serving = 1 scoop of protein powder = 25 grams of protein
- ☐ 1 serving = 4 oz (113 g) of chicken, fish = 28 grams of protein
- ☐ 1 serving = 3 oz (85 g) sirloin steak = 25 grams of protein
- ☐ 1 serving = ½ cup of egg whites = 13 grams of protein
- ☐ 1 serving = 1 oz (28 g) of low fat cheese = 7 grams of protein
- ☐ 1 serving = 1 cup of lima beans= 15 grams of protein
- ☐ 1 serving = 4 oz (113 g) of firm tofu = 10 grams of protein

When selecting your protein sources, it is best to choose those that have a lower amount of saturated fats, which means less red meat with marbled fat and more poultry, fish, and tofu. To reduce the saturated fat level of poultry even further, remove the skin and any white fat deposits before cooking.

The Truestar Way to Eat Protein

EAT:

- ☐ Lean turkey or chicken breast
- ☐ Fish and seafood: wild salmon, mackerel, haddock, halibut, sole, crab, lobster, shrimp and light tuna (avoid white tuna due to its potentially high mercury content — light tuna has significantly less mercury)
- ☐ Egg whites in a shake or omelet
- ☐ Omega-3 eggs
- ☐ Low-fat yogurt
- ☐ Skim milk (unless lactose intolerant)
- ☐ Low-fat cottage cheese or other low-fat cheeses
- ☐ Goat cheese
- ☐ Occasional lean beef or pork
- ☐ Protein powder
- ☐ Tofu veggie burgers, imitation ground beef, or tofu cheese

DON'T EAT:

- ☐ Meats high in saturated fat: beefsteak, pork ribs, and fast foods. When eaten in excess, they may also harm the heart.

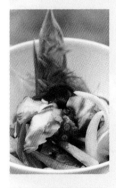

Many people are eating far too many refined carbohydrates and far too little protein. The Truestar weight loss and total health menu plans correct this imbalance.

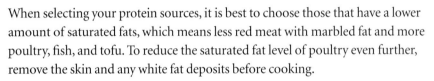

Fats

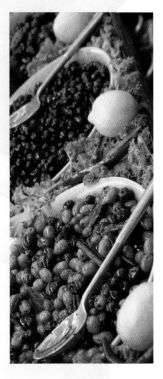

Fats are a third macronutrient that are a necessary part of every diet. Fats play a significant role in brain development, weight loss, energy levels, and protection against heart disease and stroke. In fact, 60% of the brain is comprised of fat! A lack of 'good' fats in the diet has been indicated as a major contributing factor in the development of allergies, asthma, heart disease, inflammation, arthritis, depression, and attention deficit disorder. Alternatively, an excess of 'bad' fats can lead to many of these same illnesses. Let's examine the various types of fat in the diet to decipher the good fats from the bad.

GOOD FATS, BAD FATS

There are four major categories of fats: some are good, some are bad, and some are either good or bad, depending on the amount we eat.

FOUR TYPES OF FAT

- Saturated fats
- Monounsaturated fats
- Polyunsaturated fats
- Trans fats

SATURATED FATS

These fats are found mostly in animal products (red meat), dairy products (whole milk, cream), and tropical oils, such as coconut, palm, and palm kernel oil. The liver uses saturated fats to produce necessary cholesterol, but excessive consumption of saturated fats can raise the level of the 'bad' cholesterol, known as low-density lipoprotein (LDL). Although cholesterol plays a vital role in our bodies, maintaining proper structure of our cell walls and producing the sex hormones estrogen and testosterone and the adrenal hormone cortisol, an increase in the amount of cholesterol we produce can also have detrimental effects on blood flow.

Eating large amounts of saturated fat increases the level of LDL in our system, causing stiffening and narrowing of the arterial walls. Damage to the arterial walls increases the risk of cardiovascular disease, heart attack, stroke, and other vascular disturbances. It is best to keep these fats to a minimum in the diet (approximately 5%).

MONOUNSATURATED FATS

These fats are considered to be 'good' fats. Found in olive, canola, and peanut oils, as well as in avocados, monounsaturated fats appear to lower 'bad' cholesterol (LDL) and have minimal or no effect on the 'good' cholesterol (HDL). Olive oil contains the highest amount of monounsaturated fats of all the edible oils. The best type of olive oil is labeled "extra-virgin," made from the first pressing of the olives. This oil is very flavorful and can be used for cooking or in salad dressings. Store in a dark, cool place.

These fats are found in most vegetable oils, such as soybean, corn, safflower, and sunflower oils. Although these fats have the positive effect of lowering your 'bad' cholesterol, when eaten in excess, poly-unsaturated fats (PUFAs) also have a tendency to lower your 'good' cholesterol (HDL).

Essential Fatty Acids

All fats are composed of building blocks called fatty acids. In the PUFA family, there are two types that are classified as *essential fatty acids*. These fatty acids are called essential because they are vital for health and cannot be produced by the body. Every living cell in the body needs essential fatty acids to rebuild and produce new cells.

There are two basic categories of essential fatty acids that need to be balanced in our body: omega-3 fatty acids (called alpha-linolenic acid) and omega-6 fatty acids (called linoleic acid). Too many PUFAs in the form of processed vegetable oils can create an imbalance in the ratio of omega-6 to omega-3 essential fatty acids.

The balance of omega-6 to omega-3 is very important and has a teeter-totter sort of effect. In other words, if an individual has too much of one kind, they will become deficient in the other. Most North Americans are chronically deficient in omega-3 essential fats. Allergies, eczema, inflammatory conditions

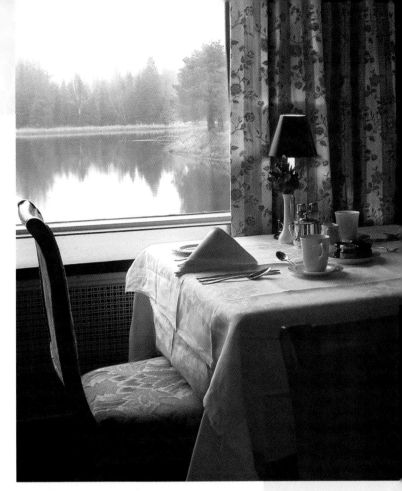

(arthritis, colitis), constipation, attention deficit disorder (ADD), and other learning disabilities have all been linked to a deficiency of this precious fat.

The ideal ratio of omega-6 to omega-3 fat is approximately 1:1, but due to the overconsumption of vegetable oils found in processed foods, the average ratio now ranges between 20:1 and 30:1. We need to eat more omega-3 and better omega-6 fatty acids.

Good sources of omega-3 fatty acids include fish oil supplements, flaxseed oil, omega-3 eggs, deep-water fish, walnuts and walnut oil, and soybeans. Optimal sources of omega-6 fatty acids include raw nuts, seeds, legumes, borage oil, grapeseed oil, and evening primrose oil.

Trans fats increase the production of 'bad' cholesterol (LDL) and decrease the production of 'good' cholesterol (HDL). They are bad for your heart, cause hardening and narrowing of the arteries, and lead to the development of type II diabetes.

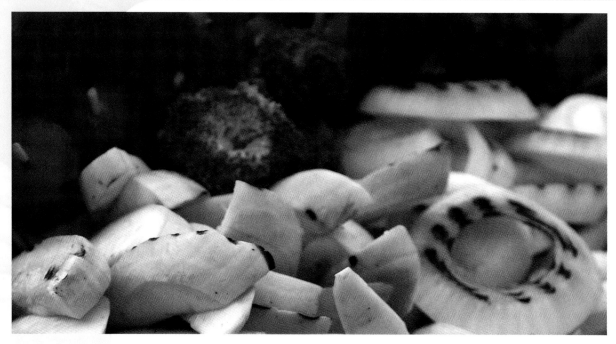

Prior to beginning any diet plan, it is best to check with your primary health-care practitioner to determine if you have any health problem that a weight-loss program might affect — and to establish an ideal or target weight for you.

These fatty acids are manufactured fats, found in margarine, snack foods, microwave popcorn, and fried foods. Food manufacturers produce trans-fatty acids (TFAs) by heating polyunsaturated vegetable oils and converting them to solid foods, such as shortening and margarine. These hydrogenated oils reduce manufacturing costs, extend storage life of a product, and can even improve flavor and texture.

Manufactured fats are extremely detrimental to health and should be eliminated from the diet completely. Trans fats increase the production of 'bad' cholesterol (LDL) and decrease the production of 'good' cholesterol (HDL). They are bad for your heart, cause hardening and narrowing of the arteries, and lead to the development of type II diabetes. In addition, when polyunsaturated fats are heated to high temperatures and become trans fats, they release free radicals, which are precursors to cancer-causing agents in your body.

Check food labels carefully — if you see the words "partially hydrogenated oils," move on. This product contains trans-fatty acids.

Sample Serving Sizes of Fats

As a general rule, the amount of 'good fat' that should be consumed daily for adult men and women is approximately 30% of total caloric intake (approximately 50-60 grams per day, 10-15 grams per meal, and 3-5 grams per snack). Of this amount, only 5% of total fat grams should be derived from saturated fat.

Recommended Servings

- 1 serving = 1 tsp of extra virgin olive oil = 5 grams of fat
- 1 serving = 7 almonds = 5 grams of fat
- 1 serving = ⅛ of an avocado = 5 grams of fat
- 1 serving = 1 tablespoon of peanut butter = 5 grams of fat

The Truestar Way of Eating Fats

EAT:

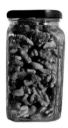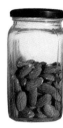

- High quality fish oils daily in supplement form
- Monounsaturated fats, such as olive oil, avocados, almonds, walnuts, sesame seeds, sunflower seeds
- Foods rich in omega-3 fats, such as cold-water fish, walnuts, and omega-3 eggs
- Omega-6 oils, such as borage oil, grapeseed oil, and evening primrose oil

DON'T EAT:

- Trans-fatty acids and partially hydrogenated oils found in margarine and other processed food items
- Deep-fried foods
- Vegetable oils, such as safflower, sunflower, and sesame oil, especially if they will be heated

Minimize saturated fat in the diet found in red meat and full-fat cheeses. These types of fats can cause inflammation and damage to the heart.

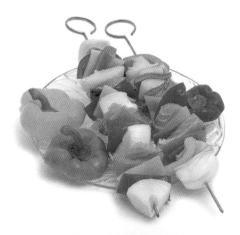

Truestar Weight Loss Plan

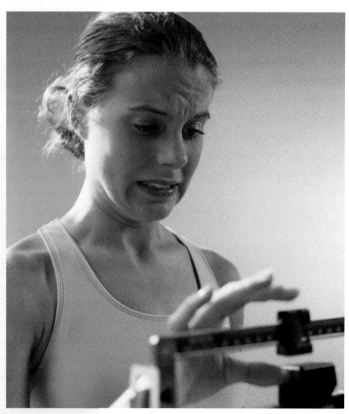

When people have a higher metabolism, they are less likely to become overweight. They are the lucky ones. Still, for the rest of us, if we boost our metabolic rate, we can lose weight.

Now that you have a basic understanding of the carbohydrate, protein, and fat components of a good diet, let's discover how Truestar's phase-based weight-loss programs can work for you!

Prior to beginning any diet plan, it is best to check with your primary health-care practitioner to determine if you have any health problem that a weight-loss program might affect — and to establish an ideal or target weight for you.

Healthy Weight

To determine an ideal weight for optimal health and lifelong fitness, health-care professionals have developed a calculation called the body mass index (BMI). The BMI was designed to alert us to how weight can put us at risk for several weight-related health conditions, such as diabetes and heart disease.

The BMI is based on a ratio of height to weight. To calculate your BMI, measure your height and weight in imperial units and trace these figures on a Body Mass Index Chart.

For the average woman, the ideal BMI is above 19.1 and below 25.8. For the average man, above 20.7 and below 26.4. Your ideal or target weight for good health should be a BMI within these ranges.

For example, if you are 66 inches tall (5 feet, 6 inches), your weight should range from 118 to 155 pounds to be in the recommended BMI range. You will want to work with health-care professionals to establish a safe and healthy target weight within this range.

Body mass index may not be accurate:

- It may overestimate body fat in athletes and others who have a muscular build.

- It may underestimate body fat in older persons and others who have lost muscle mass.

Measuring Weight Loss

At Truestar, we not only 'weigh' weight loss on a scale, we 'measure' inches lost with a ruler or tape measure.

10 Standardized Sites for Circumference Measurements

All measurements should be taken to the nearest half inch, and all measurements on the limbs should be taken on the right side of the body. Have someone take your measurements at the end of each month and chart your progress.

- Neck: Place the tape directly under the chin so that it is parallel to the floor. Apply minimal pressure as you take the measurement.

- Shoulder: Apply the tape snugly around the largest area of the shoulder muscles and take the measurement as you exhale.

- Chest: Place the tape measure over the largest area of the chest and parallel to the floor. Take the measurement from behind at the end of a normal expiration.

- Waist: Place the tape snugly over the narrowest part of the torso.

- Abdominal: This measurement is taken directly over the belly button. Make sure the tape is placed horizontally and under the clothing. Again take the measurement after a normal expiration.

- Hips: Apply the tape snugly around the largest area in the hip region. Take the measurement standing at side and make sure the tape is placed parallel to the floor.

- Thigh: Rest one foot on a chair or bench. Measure half way between the bent knee and the inguinal (the line that separates the buttocks from the upper hamstring) crease located at the top of the leg. Take the measurement at this site, placing the tape securely around the thigh.

- Calf: Rest one foot on a chair or bench, place the tape horizontally around the largest girth of the calf, and take the measurement.

- Arm: With the elbow bent to 90º but relaxed, place the tape around the arm at a level halfway between the tip of the elbow and the top of the shoulder. Take the measurement in this area facing the side of the member.

- Wrist: With the elbow bent to 90º and the palm facing up, place the tape around the wrist directly above the palm.

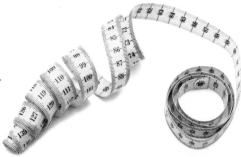

	Color
	Under-weight
	Healthy Weight
	Hefty
	Prosperous
	Grossly Prosperous

BMI

Height (in)

Weight (lbs)	58	59	60	61	62	63	64	65	66	67	68	69	70	71	72	73	74	75	76
	4'10"	4'11"	5'0"	5'1"	5'2"	5'3"	5'4"	5'5"	5'6"	5'7"	5'8"	5'9"	5'10"	5'11"	6'0"	6'1"	6'2"	6'3"	6'4"
100	21	20	20	19	18	18	17	17	16	16	15	15	14	14	14	13	13	13	12
105	22	21	21	20	19	19	18	18	17	16	16	16	15	15	14	14	14	13	13
110	23	22	22	21	20	20	19	18	18	17	17	16	16	15	15	15	14	14	13
115	24	23	23	22	21	20	20	19	19	18	18	17	17	16	16	15	15	14	14
120	25	24	23	23	22	21	21	20	19	19	18	18	17	17	16	16	15	15	15
125	26	25	24	24	23	22	22	21	20	20	19	18	18	17	17	17	16	16	15
130	27	26	25	25	24	23	22	22	21	20	20	19	19	18	18	17	17	16	16
135	28	27	26	26	25	24	23	23	22	21	21	20	19	19	18	18	17	17	16
140	29	28	27	27	26	25	24	23	23	22	21	21	20	20	19	19	18	18	17
145	30	29	28	27	27	26	25	24	23	23	22	21	21	20	20	19	19	18	18
150	31	30	29	28	27	27	26	25	24	24	23	22	22	21	20	20	19	19	18
155	32	31	30	29	28	28	27	26	25	24	24	23	22	22	21	20	20	19	19
160	34	32	31	30	29	28	28	27	26	25	24	24	23	22	22	21	21	20	20
165	35	33	32	31	30	29	28	28	27	26	25	24	24	23	22	22	21	21	20
170	36	34	33	32	31	30	29	28	27	27	26	25	24	24	23	22	22	21	21
175	37	35	34	33	32	31	30	29	28	27	27	26	25	24	24	23	23	22	21
180	38	36	35	34	33	32	31	30	29	28	27	27	26	25	24	24	23	23	22
185	39	37	36	35	34	33	32	31	30	29	28	27	27	26	25	24	24	23	23
190	40	38	37	36	35	34	33	32	31	30	29	28	27	27	26	25	24	24	23
195	41	39	38	37	36	35	34	33	32	31	30	29	28	27	27	26	25	24	24
200	42	40	39	38	37	36	34	33	32	31	30	30	29	28	27	26	26	25	24
205	43	41	40	39	38	36	35	34	33	32	31	30	29	29	28	27	26	26	25
210	44	43	41	40	38	37	36	35	34	33	32	31	30	29	29	28	27	26	26
215	45	44	42	41	39	38	37	36	35	34	33	32	31	30	29	28	28	27	26
220	46	45	43	42	40	39	38	37	36	35	34	33	32	31	30	29	28	28	27
225	47	46	44	43	41	40	39	38	36	35	34	33	32	31	31	30	29	28	27

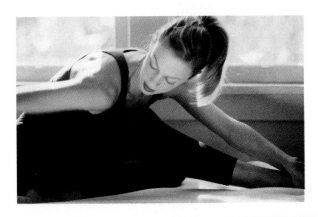

	Under-weight
	Healthy Weight
	Hefty
	Prosperous
	Grossly Prosperous

BMI

Weight (lbs)	Height (in)																		
	58	59	60	61	62	63	64	65	66	67	68	69	70	71	72	73	74	75	76
	4'10"	4'11"	5'0"	5'1"	5'2"	5'3"	5'4"	5'5"	5'6"	5'7"	5'8"	5'9"	5'10"	5'11"	6'0"	6'1"	6'2"	6'3"	6'4"
230	48	47	45	44	42	41	40	38	37	36	35	34	33	32	31	30	30	29	28
235	49	48	46	44	43	42	40	39	38	37	36	35	34	33	32	31	30	29	29
240	50	49	47	45	44	43	41	40	39	38	37	36	35	34	33	32	31	30	29
245	51	50	48	46	45	43	42	41	40	38	37	36	35	34	33	32	32	31	30
250	52	51	49	47	46	44	43	42	40	39	38	37	36	35	34	33	32	31	30
255	53	52	50	48	47	45	44	43	41	40	39	38	37	36	35	34	33	32	31
260	54	53	51	49	48	46	45	43	42	41	40	38	37	36	35	34	33	33	32
265	56	54	52	50	49	47	46	44	43	42	40	39	38	37	36	35	34	33	32
270	57	55	53	51	49	48	46	45	44	42	41	40	39	38	37	36	35	34	33
275	58	56	54	52	50	49	47	46	44	43	42	41	40	38	37	36	35	34	34
280	59	57	55	53	51	50	48	47	45	44	43	41	40	39	38	37	36	35	34
285	60	58	56	54	52	51	49	48	46	45	43	42	41	40	39	38	37	36	35
290	61	59	57	55	53	51	50	48	47	46	44	43	42	41	39	38	37	36	35
295	62	60	58	56	54	52	51	49	48	46	45	44	42	41	40	39	38	37	36
300	63	61	59	57	55	53	52	50	49	47	46	44	43	42	41	40	39	38	37

Log on to www.truestarhealth.com to create a personal nutritional meal plan based on your weight-loss goals, physical activity level, and current health status.

Metabolic Boost

All of the Truestar meal plans and recipes have been created with specific amounts of carbohydrates, proteins, and fats to help you boost your metabolism and lose weight.

Our metabolism can be thought of as the rate at which we use energy to keep our body functioning. Our body uses energy to keep the heart beating and the lungs breathing, to keep us warm and to digest food, and to allow our muscles to work. Our metabolism provides the energy for all these functions.

Some people's bodies need to use more energy to perform all necessary functions. These people are said to have a faster metabolism. When people have a faster metabolism, they are less likely to become overweight. These people are rare, however. For the rest of us, we need to eat a balanced diet to boost our metabolism and achieve our optimal weight.

Individualized Plans

The Truestar approach to weight loss recognizes that everyone is different and, therefore, has different weight-loss needs and goals. Metabolic rates, physical activity, gender, dietary likes and dislikes, current health status, previous medical conditions, and previous dieting programs all influence future weight-loss success.

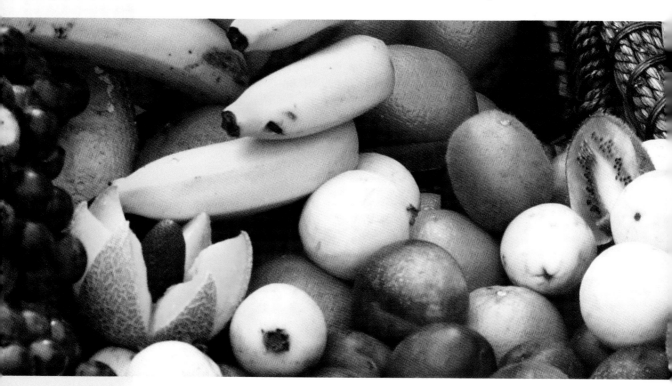

Three Phases

Truestar has developed a three-phase approach to weight loss that will fit the needs of everyone wishing to lose weight and keep it off. For example, if you want to lose weight quickly (on average, 2 to 6 pounds or more per week), Phase I: Metabolic Booster Plan has a higher protein ratio and may be most appropriate for you. If gradual weight loss is more appealing, Phase II: Continuum Weight Loss Plan is the phase for you to begin the program. To top it off, once the weight has been lost, Truestar offers a variety of Healthy Weighty Maintenance Plans that contain hundreds of delicious recipes and meal options to keep the weight off for life!

Phase I: Metabolic Booster Plan
- Average weight loss is approximately 2 to 6 pounds per week, based on the Truestar program

Phase II: Continuum Weight Loss Plan
- Average weight loss is approximately 2 pounds per week , based on the Truestar program

Phase III: Weight Loss Maintenance Plan
- Weight loss is maintained over the long-term, based on the Truestar program

NOTE: Weight loss can vary per individual. People with certain medical conditions (e.g., thyroid disorders) may lose weight at slower rates and should consult their doctor if weight-loss results are not achieved.

When people have a higher metabolism, they are less likely to become over-weight.

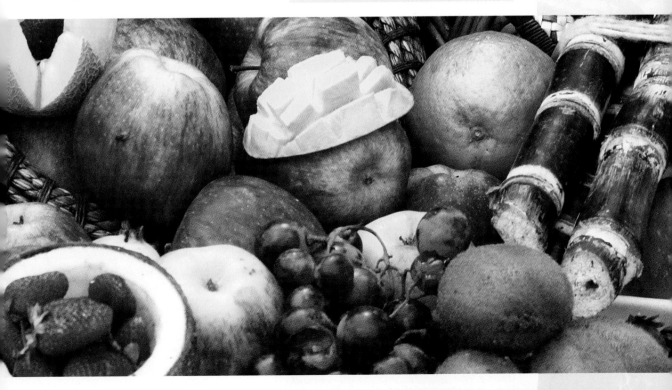

Phase I

Metabolic Booster Plan

(Lose, on average, 2 to 6 pounds per week)
The Metabolic Booster Plan is suitable for those who wish to lose weight in a quick, safe, and easy manner. On average, in the first 4 to 6 weeks, you can expect to lose a minimum of 2 to 6 pounds per week. In subsequent weeks, an average weight loss of 1 to 2 pounds per week is normal. Weight loss can vary, however.

This plan is best suited for those who have trouble with blood sugar control, who have a slow metabolism, or are chronic dieters with difficulty losing weight. For example, individuals who have been diagnosed with type II diabetes, insulin resistance, hypoglycemia

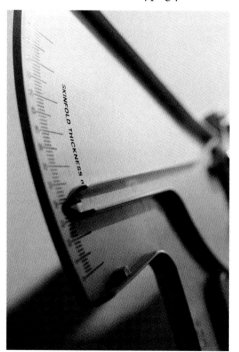

(low blood sugar), high blood pressure, high cholesterol, obesity, and heart disease would do best on this plan. People with certain medical conditions, such as thyroid disorders, may lose weight at slower rates and should consult their doctor if weight loss results are not achieved.

For optimal weight loss results and to rev up your metabolism permanently, it is best to stay on the metabolic booster phase for a minimum of 6 weeks. For certain conditions, such as type II diabetes and hypoglycemia, the metabolic booster phase is appropriate for long-term use. If you experience weight gain when switching over to Phase II: Continuum Weight Loss Plan, it is likely that your blood sugar response is not yet under control, and you are still secreting too much insulin, with excess sugar being stored as fat. To continue to regulate and boost your metabolism, simply return to the Phase I: Metabolic Booster Plan for a 4- to 6-week period.

Metabolic Booster Food Ratio

To boost your metabolism, you need to eat a specific ratio of carbohydrates, proteins, and fats.

- ☐ 40% lean proteins
- ☐ 30% low glycemic index carbohydrates
- ☐ 30% essential fats

You need to eat in this ratio, approximately, for each and every meal and snack in order to lose your desired weight.

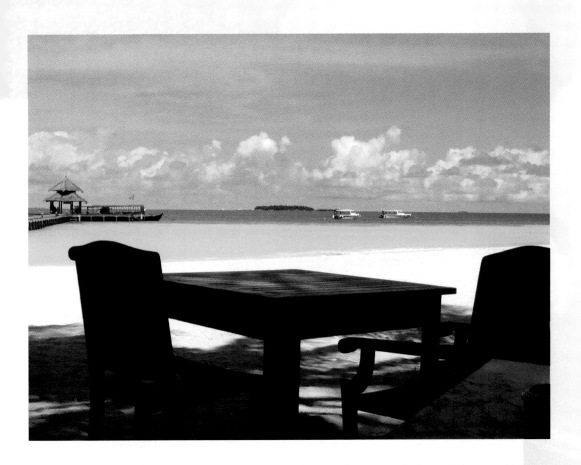

Common Food Measurements and Conversion Tables
Measuring Liquids

CUPS	OZ	ML
1 dash	6 drops	0.4 ml
24 drops	¼ tsp	1.2 ml
3 tsp	1 tbsp	14 ml
1 tbsp	½ oz	14 ml
2 tbsp	1 oz	29 ml
3 tbsp (1 jigger)	1½ ounces	44 ml
½ cup	4 oz	118 ml
16 tbsp	1 cup	237 ml
1 cup (½ pint)	8 oz	237 ml
2 cups (1 pint)	16 oz	474 ml
4 cups (1 quart)	32 oz	946 ml

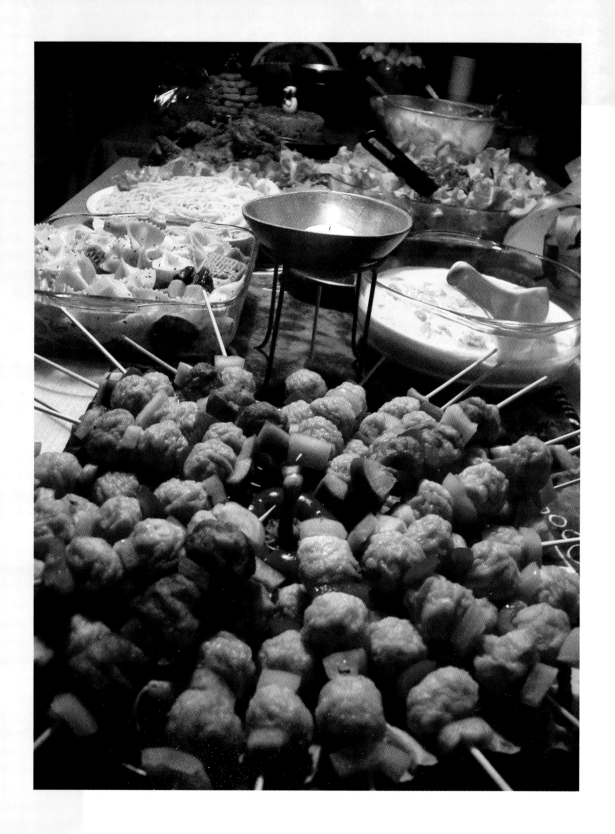

Protein Factor

The protein proportion is slightly higher in the Metabolic Booster Plan in order to jump start metabolism and shed extra fat storage.

The hormone glucagon is released in response to dietary protein. Glucagon signals fat cells to release their fat into the blood, thereby promoting its use. In other words, more fat is burned and more weight is lost when protein is increased.

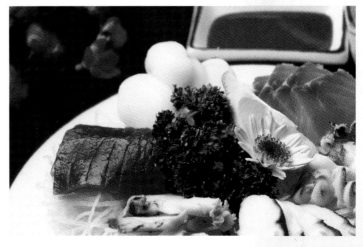

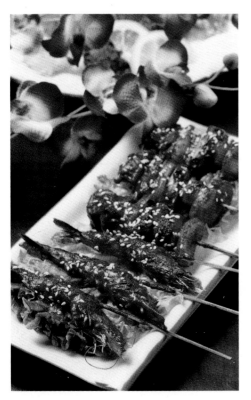

Meal Plans

If you are eating directly from the Truestar meal plans, you need not worry — all of the meals are precisely balanced according to you!

RESTRICTED AND ALLOWED FOODS

In the Metabolic Booster Plan, high glycemic index and high glycemic load foods, as well as certain proteins and fats, are restricted, while others are allowed.

More fat is burned and more weight is lost when protein is increased.

Metabolic Booster Plan: Carbohydrates Restricted

Fruits	*Vegetables*	*Refined Flours*	*Sugars and Alcohol*
• Grapes	• White potatoes	• Cereals	• Candy
• Raisins	• Sweet potatoes	• Instant oatmeal	• Ice cream
• Cranberries	• White rice	• White bread, buns, bagels	• Granola bars
• Dates	• Squash	• Pasta	• Beer, wine, liquor
• Fruit juices		• Crackers and Cookies	• Soda/pop

Carbohydrates Allowed

Fruits	*Vegetables*	*Beans*	*Whole Grains*
• Apples	• Broccoli	• Navy beans	• 2 pieces Wasa crisps
• Apricots	• Spinach	• Kidney beans	• 1 cup of slow cooking oatmeal
• Bananas (1 small)	• Tomatoes	• Black beans	• 1 medium-sized whole-wheat tortilla wrap
• Cherries	• Tomato sauce	• Lentils	
• Grapefruit	• Cauliflower	• Chick peas	
• Oranges	• Peppers	• Mung beans	
• Nectarines	• Green beans	• Pinto beans	
• Peaches	• Mushrooms	• Romano beans	
• Pears	• Water chestnuts	• Soy beans	
• Plums	• Romaine lettuce	• Garbanzo beans	
• Prunes (pitted)	• Radicchio	• Chick peas	
• Raspberries	• Onions	• Split peas	
• Strawberries	• Zucchini		
• Blueberries	• Cucumber		
• Blackberries	• Kale		
• Watermelon	• Cabbage		
	• Collard greens		
	• Bok choy		

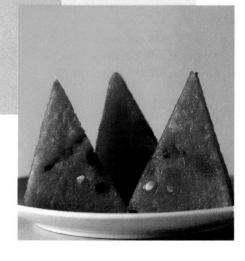

Metabolic Booster Plan: Proteins Restricted	Proteins Allowed
• Full-fat cheeses • Fatty meat products: beefsteak, pork ribs 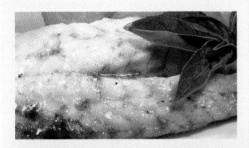	Low-fat dairy products: 1% or skim milk, low-fat yogurt, cottage cheese, cheese Omega-3 eggs and egg whites Protein powder Soy products: fortified soy milk, soy meats, soy cheese, tofu, miso, veggie burgers Chicken breast, slices, ground chicken Turkey slices, turkey bacon, turkey breast, ground turkey Lean ground beef and lean beef and veal Fish: salmon, tuna, mackerel, cod, anchovies, sardines, halibut, sole
Metabolic Booster Plan: Fats Restricted	Fats Allowed
• Deep-fried foods: potato chips, French fries • Full-fat cheese • Fat-marbled meats • Partially hydrogenated food items • Hydrogenated margarine (check label) • Vegetable oils: safflower, sunflower	Ground flaxseeds or flaxseed oil Nuts and seeds: almonds, walnuts, soy nuts, cashews, sesame seeds (½ handful daily) Avocado (¼ daily) Non-hydrogenated margarine Butter (sparingly) Extra-virgin olive oil, olives (black or green) Almond, avocado, canola, pumpkin, soybean, borage, fish oil (supplements)

Log on to www.truestarhealth.com to create a personal nutritional meal plan based on your weight-loss goals, physical activity level, and current health status.

Sample Metabolic Booster Meal Plans and Recipes

When adding fat to your meal or snack, try 'sprinkling' good fats on your food — topping a salad with crushed walnuts, adding flax oil to a morning shake, or using olive oil for cooking. Fat has nearly twice as many calories as protein and carbohydrates, so you don't need as much to reap all the benefits.

Remember to combine a selection of carbohydrates, protein, and fat at each and every meal and snack. Truestar recipes include a measure of the total carbohydrates, proteins, and fats in each recipe so you can quickly see if the desired macronutrient ratio is being met. While the ideal ratio cannot always be met, aim to keep the proportions close to the ideal.

These are only a few elementary recipes that combine all three macronutrients (carbohydrates, proteins, and fats). Truestar has created thousands of easy-to-prepare meal and snack recipes, featuring hormonally balanced foods choices that promote a lifetime of healthy eating and weight loss.

For more Metabolic Booster Plan recipes, see the Truestar Recipes section in this book and the truestarhealth.com website.

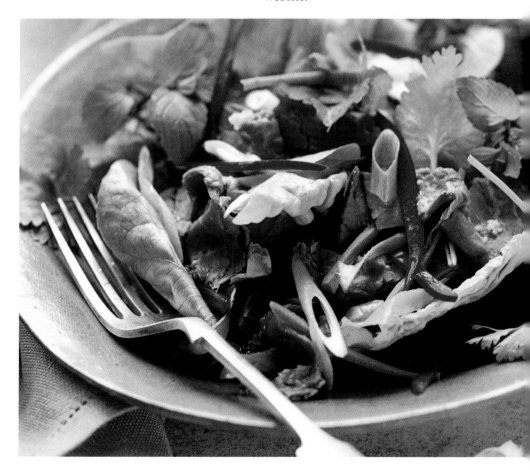

Banana Raspberry Smoothie

- 6¼ tbsp (30 grams) protein powder
- 4 oz (118 ml) soy milk
- ¼ medium banana
- ½ cup frozen raspberries
- 1½ cup (7 ml) flaxseed oil

Blend on high and enjoy!

MACRONUTRIENT RATIO

- Carbohydrates: 23 grams
- Protein: 26 grams
- Fat: 10 grams

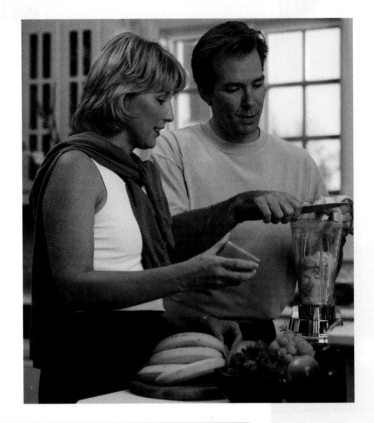

Mediterranean Beef Salad

- 5 oz (142 g) lean eye of round beef
- 2 cups romaine lettuce
- ½ cup sliced red pepper
- ¾ cup chopped onion
- ½ cup sliced mushrooms
- 1½ tsp (7.4 ml) extra-virgin olive oil
- ⅛ tsp (0.6 ml) Worcestershire sauce
- 2 tsp (9.8 ml) red table wine
- ½ tsp (2.3 g) minced garlic

Combine oil, thinly sliced beef, peppers, mushrooms, onion, Worcestershire sauce, garlic, and red wine in a nonstick pan. Cook until beef is browned and pepper and onions are tender. Cover and simmer for 5 minutes until mixture is hot, stirring occasionally to blend flavors. Arrange garden salad mix of romaine lettuce on a large plate. Spoon beef and vegetable mixture onto top of salad. Sprinkle with salt and pepper. Enjoy!

MACRONUTRIENT RATIO

Carbohydrates: 26 grams • Protein: 32 grams • Fat: 12 grams

Sweet and Sour Chicken

- 5 oz (142 g) boneless, skinless chicken breast
- 2.5 tsp (12 ml) extra-virgin olive oil
- ¼ cup (57 g) raw snow peas
- ½ cup (114 g)raw onions
- ¼ cup (57 g) mung bean sprouts
- ¼ cup (57 g) pineapple wedges
- 2 tsp (9.9 ml) sweet and sour sauce

Heat half the oil in a nonstick pan over medium-high heat. Add pieces of chicken and cook for approximately 10 minutes or until chicken is no longer pink inside. Coat another nonstick pan with remaining oil and heat over medium-high heat. Add snow peas, onions, and sprouts. Sauté until crisp yet tender. Mix in pineapple and sweet and sour sauce. Cook an additional 3 to 5 minutes. Place on a plate and top with chicken.

MACRONUTRIENT RATIO
Carbohydrates: 46 g • Protein: 47 g • Fat: 14 g

Phase II

NOTE: Weight loss can vary per individual. People with certain medical conditions (e.g., thyroid disorders) may lose weight at slower rates and should consult their doctor if weight-loss results are not achieved.

Continuum Weight Loss Plan

(Lose 1 to 2 pounds per week)
The Continuum Weight Loss Plan is designed for individuals who have successfully completed the Metabolic Booster Plan (4 to 6 weeks) and wish to eat more whole grains and carbohydrates in their diet or for those who desire a more gradual weight-loss approach. On Phase II, you can expect to lose weight at approximately 1 to 2 pounds per week.

Once you have successfully completed Phase I, your metabolism should be working at a faster pace and you should not gain any weight when switching to Phase II. If you do find yourself gaining weight, simply switch back to the Metabolic Booster Plan for another 4- to 6-week period.

Continuum Weight Loss Food Ratio

In this phase, you need to eat a slightly different ratio of carbohydrates, proteins, and fats, with an increase in carbohydrates.

- 40% low glycemic index carbohydrates (10% higher than the Metabolic Booster Plan)
- 30% lean proteins (10% less than the Metabolic Booster Plan)
- 30% essential fats

You need to eat in this ratio for each and every meal and snack in order to continue losing your weight.

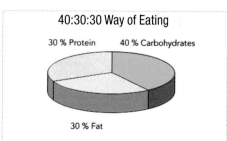

40:30:30 Way of Eating

30 % Protein   40 % Carbohydrates

30 % Fat

The foods allowed in the Continuum Weight Loss Plan are similar to the Metabolic Booster Plan, but there is a higher percentage of carbohydrates, especially whole-grain items. Additionally, four alcoholic beverages per week are permitted. Optimal choices are red wine or light beer. Be sure to have a selection of protein if indulging in alcoholic beverages.

Restricted and allowed proteins and fats are the same as for the Metabolic Booster Plan. Eat fatty meat products, such as beefsteak and pork ribs, minimally, once a week only, and avoid full-fat cheeses, eating instead low-fat cheddar, mozzarella, havarti, and other cheeses.

Continuum Weight Loss Plan: Carbohydrates Allowed

Fruits	Vegetables	Beans	Whole Grains
• All fruits with the exception of dates, raisins, and sugary juices	• All vegetables are allowed except for white potatoes. • Sweet potatoes and squash are allowed	• All types of beans, legumes, and seeds	• 2 pieces crispbread • 1 cup of slow cooking oatmeal • 1 medium-sized whole-wheat tortilla wrap • ½ cup of kamut or spelt pasta • ½ cup of brown rice • 2 slices of whole-grain bread

Carbohydrates Restricted

Fruits	Vegetables	Sugar	Refined Flour
• Fruit juice	• White potatoes or rice	• Candy and ice cream • Granola bars • Soda/pop	• White pasta, white bagels, crackers, and cookies • Cereals and instant oatmeal • White bread and buns (aside from Wasa crispbread)

Meal Plans

Truestar meal plans and recipes are balanced precisely to normalize insulin levels. The whole grains found in our meal plans are made of rich fibers and flours, such as kamut and spelt pasta or multi-grain and flaxseed bread.

Remember, the key is to balance the three macronutrients at the ratio we recommend. Eating carbohydrates, proteins, and fats separate from each other is *not* the key to weight loss.

Once you have lost your desired weight, if you eat whole grains in moderation and in combination with the proper amounts of protein and fat, the weight you have lost should be easily maintained. By simply

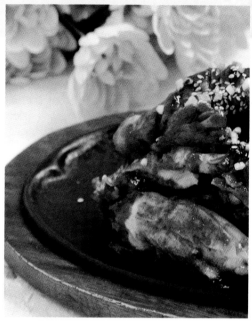

sticking to the Truestar meal plans or following our foods restricted and unrestricted — your weight loss should be permanent.

Sample Continuum Meal Plans and Recipes

BREAKFAST

Chocolate Monkey Smoothie

- 20 grams protein powder
- 8 oz (227 g) soymilk
- 3 tbsp (42 g) unsweetened cocoa powder
- ¼ banana
- 1 tsp (5 ml) flaxseed oil

Place all ingredients in a blender and blend until smooth.

MACRONUTRIENT RATIO

- Carbohydrates: 32 g
- Protein: 28 g
- Fat: 10 g

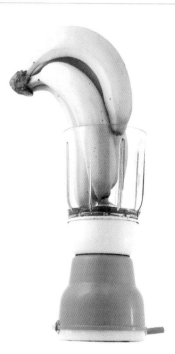

Salmon Burger and Salad

BURGER

- 5 oz (142 g) canned boneless pink salmon
- 4 tbsp (56 g) green beans
- 1/2 tsp (2.3 g) chopped chives
- 1 sweet potato boiled (small)
- 1/8 tsp (0.6 g) cayenne pepper
- salt and pepper (to taste)

In a bowl combine chopped beans, chives, salmon, mashed potato, salt, cayenne pepper and black pepper. Form mixture into a patty and grill in a nonstick pan until patties are cooked.

SALAD

2 cups lettuce
1/2 cup (142 g) cucumber
2 slices tomato
1 tbsp (14 ml) balsamic vinegar
1 tsp (5 ml) olive oil

Toss salad ingredients and serve on the side.

MACRONUTRIENT RATIO
Carbohydrates: 38 g • Protein: 31 g • Fat: 8 g

With 9 calories per gram, fat contains nearly 2.2 times the amount of calories in comparison to proteins and carbohydrates, which contain 4 calories per gram.

Feta Turkey Burger

- 3 oz (85 g) lean ground turkey
- 1 tbsp (14 g) feta cheese
- 1/2 tsp (2 ml) oregano
- ground black pepper (to taste)
- 2 cups lettuce
- 1/2 cup cucumber
- 2 slices tomato
- 1 tbsp (15 ml) balsamic vinegar
- 1 tsp (5 ml) extra-virgin olive oil
- 1 whole grain bun

Preheat grill or broiler on medium high heat. In a bowl, mix turkey, feta, oregano, and pepper. Form into a patty. Lightly oil grate and place patty onto grill. Cook for about 10 minutes or until turkey is cooked through, flipping halfway through. Place on a whole grain bun. Enjoy with tossed salad lettuce, cucumber, tomato, balsamic vinegar, olive oil).

MACRONUTRIENT RATIO
Carbohydrates: 27 g • Protein: 27 g • Fat: 10 g

Log on to www.truestarhealth.com to create a personal nutritional meal plan based on your weight-loss goals, physical activity level, and current health status.

Phase III: Healthy Weight Maintenance Plan

You should stay on the Continuum Weight Loss Plan until you reach your weight goal. Once your weight loss goal has been achieved, you can eat from any of the Truestar maintenance meal plans to keep your weight off permanently. Continue eating hormonally balanced meals not only to keep lean and fit —but also to keep your immune system strong so you can ward off any illnesses or diseases, such as diabetes, heart disease, stroke, or cancer.

Healthy Weight Maintenance Food Ratio

The food ratio for the Weight Loss Maintenance Plan is similar to Phase II, though you can introduce additional whole-grain foods to the point where you are no longer losing weight and no longer gaining weight. Keep the ratio of macronutrients for each meal and snack balanced.

- ☐ 40% low glycemic index carbohydrates
- ☐ 30% lean proteins
- ☐ 30% essential fats

In this state of metabolic balance, you should find yourself feeling fit and vital, with plenty of energy and no undue fatigue.

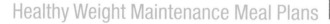

Healthy Weight Maintenance Meal Plans

The Truestar maintenance meal plans focus on nutrient-rich and delicious food options that will tempt all palates. Visit www.truestarhealth to learn more. At this site, members can fill out a personal nutritional profile to receive meal plan options that fit their lifestyle, taste buds, height, weight, and sex. There are also several customized meal plan programs available.

- ☐ Optimal wellness plans
- ☐ Red meat free plans
- ☐ Dairy free plans
- ☐ Dairy free and wheat free plans
- ☐ Gluten free plans
- ☐ Nut free plans
- ☐ Vegetarian plans
- ☐ Vegan plans

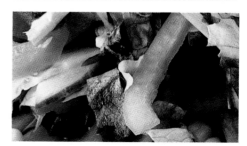

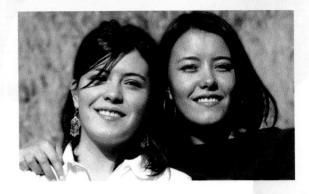

Cheating

Within the Truestar approach to eating, we have developed a cheat system that allows you to indulge occasionally in the 'no-no' foods that are typically not recommended. We call this the '80-20' rule of eating. In other words, if you follow the Truestar approach to eating 80% of the time, but fall off the health wagon and indulge 20% of the time (at parties, on weekends, or over the holiday season), you will still be able to reach and maintain your health goals.

There are three exceptions to this rule: if you are suffering from an illness or food allergy, we may advise you to follow the meal plan strictly; if you are in the first 4 weeks of the Metabolic Booster Plan; or if you are not losing any weight.

Eating for Success Guidelines

In addition to eating the proper balance of the three macronutrients at each and every meal to maintain hormonal balance, there are certain behavior and eating patterns that actually promote weight loss and optimal health. Read on to discover further tips to boost your metabolism and maintain your fit, lean, and trim body.

- ☐ Chew your food properly to avoid undigested food particles in your system. Undigested food particles are perceived as invaders in the body and can elicit an immune system attack, which can show up as digestive problems, inflammation, asthma, allergies, and poor skin.

- ☐ Take your time when eating and relax! It takes a minimum of 20 minutes for the stretch receptors in the stomach to register a 'full' or satiated signal in the brain. For this reason, eating slowly prevents overeating.

- ☐ Support optimal digestion by including plenty of fresh, clean water and fiber-filled foods in your diet.

- ☐ Do not skip meals, including breakfast. Recent research shows that people who skip meals are more likely to gain weight.

- ☐ Shop in the exterior lanes of your supermarket first, where you'll find fresh, whole foods, such as fruits, vegetables, low-fat dairy products, lean meats, and omega-3 eggs. Avoid the interior of the store, where processed food products, such as cookies, cakes, granola bars, and sugar-coated cereals, are located.

- ☐ Follow the Truestar nutrition, exercise, vitamin, attitude, and sleep programs to gain the synergistic effect of total health and weight loss the Truestar way.

- ☐ Once you begin following the Truestar approach to eating, you will notice a difference in energy and pounds lost in the first week. Within 4 weeks, you will be well on the path to a new you. Bravo — enjoy your journey on the path to the Ultimate You.

> We have developed a cheat system that allows you to indulge occasionally in the 'no-no' foods that are typically not recommended.

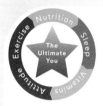

Truestar Recipes
Metabolic Booster Meal Plans

Quick and Easy Scrambled Eggs

- 2 large omega-3 eggs
- 1 large egg white
- 1 oz (28 g) non-fat dairy cheese (shredded)
- 2 tbsp (10 ml) skim milk
- 1 slice of crisp bread
- ½ cup (114 g) blueberries

Blend and cook mixture of eggs, egg whites, and shredded cheese on high heat for 1 to 1½ minutes. Enjoy with fresh fruit and crispbread on the side.

Carbohydrates 22 g • Protein: 27 g • Fat: 10 g

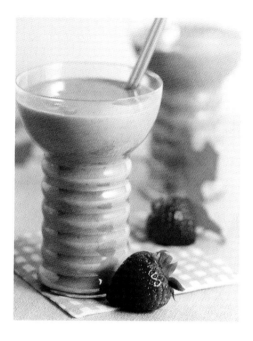

Strawberry Banana Smoothie

- ½ cup (118 ml) bananas and strawberries
- 1 scoop (25 grams) protein powder
- crushed ice
- 1 teaspoon (5 ml) flaxseed oil
- 4 oz (113 g) soymilk (added protein)

Blend on high.

Carbohydrates: 20 g • Protein: 29 g • Fat: 7 g

Cottage Cheese with Fruit Medley

- 8 oz (227 g) cottage cheese (1% fat)
- ¼ cup grapefruit
- ¼ cup mandarin orange sections
- ½ cup chopped apples
- 2 tbsp chopped almonds

Mix fruit and cheese together. Add cinnamon and nutmeg to taste if desired.

Carbohydrates: 26 g • Protein: 30 g • Fat: 10 g

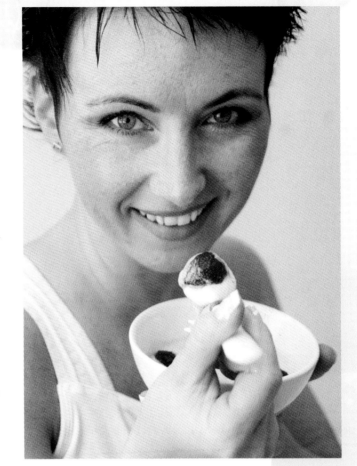

Berry Flax Yogurt

- ½ cup (115 g) low-fat, plain yogurt
- 0.7 oz (20 g) protein powder
- ¼ cup raspberries
- ¼ cup blueberries
- 1 tsp (5 ml) flaxseed oil
- 1 oz (28 ml) low-fat cheese

Mix yogurt with protein powder, flaxseed oil and berries. Serve with cheese on the side.

Carbohydrates: 22 g • Protein: 27 g • Fat: 9 g

Scrambled Eggs with Dill and Smoked Salmon

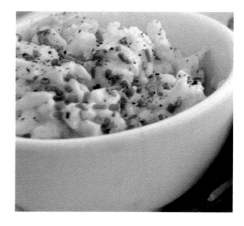

- 1 large omega-3 egg
- 3 large egg whites
- 1 tsp (5 ml) skim milk
- 1 tsp (5 g) dried dill weed
- ½ medium raw onion
- 1½ oz (42 g) smoked salmon
- 3 slices Wasa fiber crispbread
- salt (to taste)

In a large bowl, beat egg, egg whites, milk, dill, and salt. Spray a skillet with non-fat cooking oil spray. At medium heat, add sliced scallions and cook for about 8 minutes, until softened. Pour in egg mixture and cook 3 to 4 minutes, stirring occasionally, until almost set. Mix in sliced salmon. Cook 1 minute more or until eggs reach desired doneness. Enjoy with crispbread on the side.

Carbohydrates: 26 g • Protein: 30 g • Fat: 10 g

Anti-Aging Smoothie

- 1.2 oz (35 g) protein powder
- ¾ cup (177 ml) low-fat soymilk
- ½ cup whole strawberries
- ¼ cup blueberries
- 1 tbsp (15 ml) flaxseed oil
- 4 ice cubes

Blend on high and enjoy!

Carbohydrates: 29 g • Protein: 36 g • Fat: 11 g

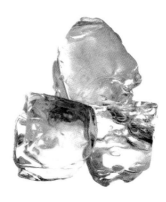

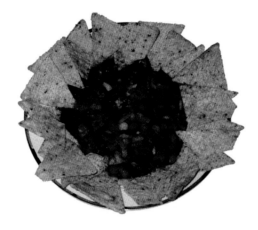

Tasty Tuna Melt

- 1 slice of whole wheat or spelt bread
- 4 oz (113 g) canned light tuna
- 1 tbsp (15 g) diced celery
- 3 slices tomato
- 1½ tsp (7 ml) light mayonnaise
- 1 oz (28 g) low-fat shredded cheese

Mix tuna, celery, tomato, mayonnaise, and cheese in a bowl. Spread mixture on bread and cook in microwave until cheese is melted on top. Enjoy with a handful of nuts!

Carbohydrates: 26 g • Protein: 40 g • Fat: 13 g

Nacho Lunch

- 15 baked nacho chips
- ⅓ cup (75 g) veggie ground beef
- 2 oz (57 g) low-fat shredded cheese
- 4 tbsp (60 ml) medium salsa

In a small baking dish, layer tortilla chips with ground beef soy, salsa, and shredded cheese. Place in microwave and cook until cheese is melted and mixture is heated (approximately 2 minutes).

Carbohydrates: 27 g • Protein: 35 g • Fat: 12 g

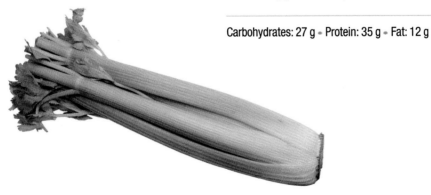

Strawberry and Pear Cottage Cheese Delight

- 1¼ cup (287 g) cottage cheese (2% fat)
- ½ cup strawberries
- ½ pear (small)
- 1½ tbsp (18 g) chopped walnuts

Combine fruit and cottage cheese. Sprinkle with nuts and enjoy!

Carbohydrates: 26 g • Protein: 42 g • Fat: 12 g

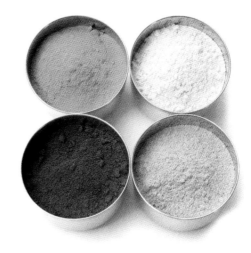

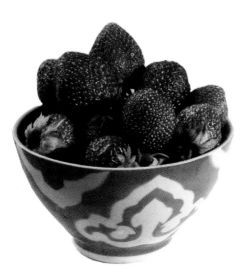

Easy Egg Salad

- 2 large hard boiled eggs
- 1 tbsp (15 ml) non-fat mayonnaise
- 1 tsp (5 ml) Dijon mustard
- 2 tbsp (28 g) diced celery
- 2½ oz (70 g) non-fat cheese
- 3 slices Wasa bread

Chop omega-3 hard-boiled eggs. In a large bowl, mix eggs with mayonnaise, mustard, and a dash of salt and pepper. Stir in chopped celery. Place cheese on crispbread and top with egg mixture.

Carbohydrates: 30 g • Protein: 36 g • Fat: 13 g

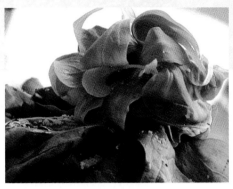

Tossed Chicken Salad

- 4 oz (113 g) cooked skinless chicken breast
- 2 oz (57 g) low-fat cheddar or colby cheese
- 1 tbsp (15 g) sunflower seeds
- 4 cups lettuce
- 1 cup cucumber
- 4 slices tomato
- 2 tbsp (30 ml) balsamic vinegar

Slice or dice chicken. Cube cheese. In a bowl, combine chicken, salad (lettuce, cucumber, tomato, and balsamic vinegar), and cubed cheese. Toss until thoroughly combined and sprinkle with sunflower seeds.

Carbohydrates: 28 g • Protein: 37 g • Fat: 12 g

Tasty Veggie Burger and Side Salad

- 1 veggie burger patty
- 1 whole wheat hamburger bun
- 1 oz (28 g) low-fat cheese shredded
- 2 tbsp sunflower seeds
- 2 cups lettuce
- ½ cup cucumber
- 2 slices tomato
- 1 tbsp balsamic vinegar
- 1 tsp (5 ml) extra-virgin olive oil
- ½ cup (115 g) low-fat yogurt
- 1 tsp ground flaxseeds

Prepare veggie burger as per package instructions. Serve with a tossed salad (lettuce, cucumber, tomato, balsamic vinegar, and olive oil). Sprinkle with sunflower seeds and shredded cheese on top. Enjoy yogurt mixed with flaxseed for dessert.

Carbohydrates: 41 g • Protein: 32 g • Fat: 13 g

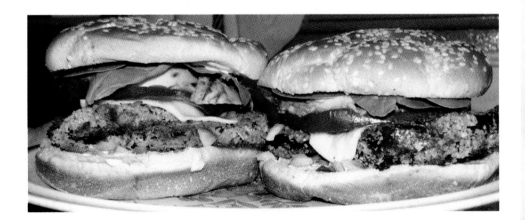

Broiled Halibut Steak with Yams and Asparagus

- 5 oz (142 g) halibut steak
- 5 medium spears of raw asparagus
- ³/₄ cup baked or broiled yams
- ¹/₂ tsp (2.3 g) paprika
- ¹/₃ tsp (1.4 g) ground oregano
- ¹/₃ tsp (1.4 g) dried thyme
- ¹/₄ tsp (1.2 g) garlic
- ¹/₈ tsp (0.125 g) cayenne pepper
- 2 tsp (9.5 g) extra-virgin olive oil

Preheat the oven to broiler setting. Combine paprika, thyme, oregano, onion powder, garlic powder, and cayenne pepper in a bowl. Mix well. Place halibut steak on a nonstick pan coated with non-fat vegetable oil spray. Brush olive oil over halibut steak. Sprinkle ¹/₂ to 1 teaspoon of seasoning mixture (use more, if desired) on top of steak. Broil for 10 minutes per inch of thickness or until fish flakes easily with a fork. Add salt and pepper to taste. Keep remaining seasoning mixture and use for next time. Serve with steamed asparagus and baked or broiled yams.

Carbohydrates: 31 g • Protein: 35 g • Fat: 12 g

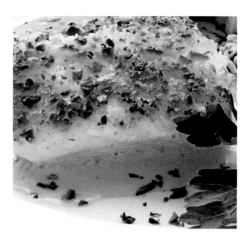

Greek Chicken Salad

- 3 cups romaine lettuce
- 7 oz (200 g) skinless chicken breast
- ¹/₂ cup (118 g) chopped tomato
- ¹/₂ cup (118 g) raw onions
- ¹/₂ cup (118 g) sliced cucumber
- ¹/₂ oz (14 g) feta cheese
- 6 black-pitted olives sliced
- 1 tbsp (14 g) extra-virgin olive oil
- 1 tbsp (15 ml) balsamic vinaigrette

Grill chicken in the oven broiler or on a barbecue. Mix lettuce, tomatoes, sliced onions, cucumbers, and olives in a large bowl. Top with sliced grilled chicken, cheese, and salad dressing made of olive oil and balsamic vinaigrette.

Carbohydrates: 33 g • Protein: 45 g • Fat: 15 g

Sunflower Tuna Salad

- 5 oz (141 g) light canned tuna
- 4 cups romaine lettuce
- ½ cup (114 g) chopped tomatoes
- ½ cup (114 g) chopped cucumber
- 2 tbsp (28 g) balsamic vinaigrette
- 1 tsp (5 ml) extra-virgin olive oil
- 1 cup cubed cantaloupe

Put all ingredients into a salad bowl and drizzle with dressing (olive oil and balsamic vinegar). Enjoy with 1 cup of cubed cantaloupe for dessert.

Carbohydrates: 33 g • Protein: 37 g • Fat: 10 g

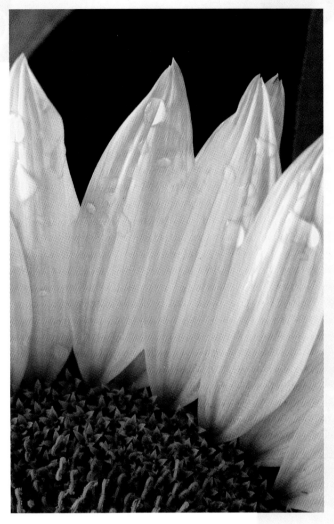

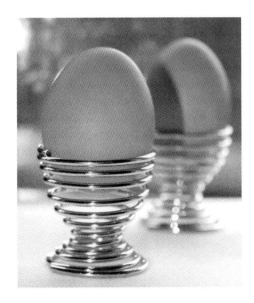

Egg Salad Crisp

- 2 large hard-boiled eggs
- 3 slices fiber crispbread
- 2 oz (57 g) non-fat cheddar cheese
- 1 tbsp (15 ml) non-fat mayonnaise

In a bowl, chop hard-boiled eggs and mix with mayonnaise. Add salt and pepper to taste. Place on top of crispbread with a slice of cheese.

Carbohydrates: 29 g • Protein: 32 g • Fat: 12 g

Grilled Teriyaki Tofu with Salad

- 3 tbsp (14 ml) teriyaki sauce
- 6 oz (120 g) low-fat firm tofu
- 2 oz (57 g) tofu cheese (mozzarella flavored)
- ½ tsp (2.3 g) dried sunflower seed kernels
- 2 cups (460 g) lettuce
- ½ cup (114 g) cucumber
- 2 slices tomato
- 1 tbsp (15 ml) balsamic vinegar
- 1 tsp (5 ml) olive oil

Cut tofu into pieces and combine with teriyaki sauce in a bowl and marinate for 20 minutes. Grill tofu, occasionally basting with extra sauce. Serve with a tossed side salad (lettuce, cucumber, tomato, balsamic vinegar, olive oil) topped with cheese and sunflower seeds. Enjoy with 2 pieces of crispbread on the side.

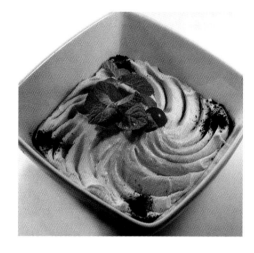

Snacks Options

- Hummus (chick pea dip) and carrots
- Yogurt and a handful of nuts
- Cottage cheese and raspberries or blueberries
- Zone protein bars
- Sliced chicken or turkey with celery and carrots
- Protein shake

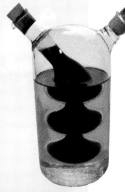

Carbohydrates: 35 g • Protein: 43 g • Fat: 11 g

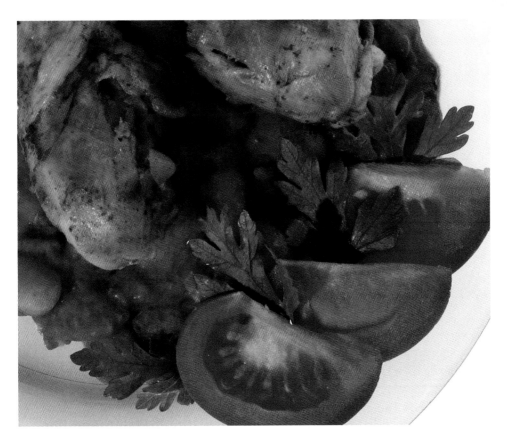

Herb Roasted Lemon Chicken

- 6 oz (170 g) raw boneless chicken breast
- ¼ medium lemon
- 2 tsp (10 g) chopped walnuts
- 1 small baked sweet potato
- 2 cups lettuce
- ½ cup (114 g) cucumber
- 2 slices tomato
- 1 tbsp (5 ml) balsamic vinegar
- 1 tsp (5 ml) olive oil

Preheat oven to 425°F. Season both sides of chicken with salt, pepper, dried rosemary, and basil. Spray baking dish with olive oil cooking spray and place chicken breast inside. Cover chicken with 2 sliced lemons and roast until chicken is no longer pink inside (about 20 minutes). Bake or microwave sweet potato at the same time. Toss salad. Enjoy!

Carbohydrates: 28 g • Protein: 41 g • Fat: 12 g

Continuum Weight Loss Meal Plans

Ham and Cheese Omelet

- 1 large omega-3 egg
- 1 large egg white
- 1 oz (28 g) extra lean ham
- 1 oz (28 g) low-fat cheddar cheese
- ½ tsp (2.5 ml) olive oil
- 1 orange
- 1 kiwi

Spray a nonstick pan with cooking oil spray and heat over medium heat. In a bowl, whisk together egg and egg whites. Pour into pan and add chopped ham and shredded cheese. When eggs are set, flip over and continue cooking until egg is fully cooked. Serve with fruit.

Carbohydrates: 29 g • Protein: 24 g • Fat: 10 g

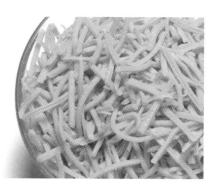

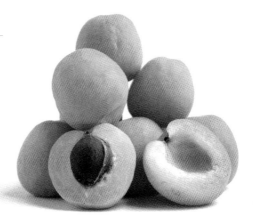

Apricot Power Oatmeal

- ½ cup (115 g) oatmeal cereal
- 8 fl oz (236 ml) water
- 1 scoop protein powder
- 1 tbsp (5 g) dried apricots
- ⅛ tsp (0.5 g) ground cinnamon
- 1½ tbsp (21 g) chopped almonds

Prepare slow-cooking oatmeal following package instructions. Mix protein powder into a small amount of soymilk or water. Mix into prepared oatmeal. Add chopped apricot, cinnamon, and nuts.

Carbohydrates: 25 g • Protein: 20 g • Fat: 8 g

Immune-Boosting Smoothie

- 2 tbsp (30 g) protein powder
- 8 fl oz (236 ml) filtered water
- ¼ cup orange sherbet
- 1 cup whole strawberries
- ¼ banana
- 1½ tsp (7 ml) flaxseed oil

Place fruit, water, protein powder, flaxseed oil, and sherbet in a blender. Blend until smooth. Enjoy.

Carbohydrates: 30 g • Protein: 23 g • Fat: 10 g

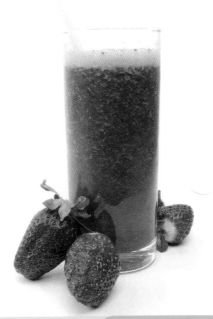

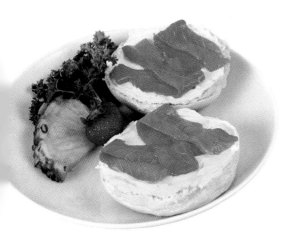

Bagel, Cream Cheese, and Smoked Salmon (Lox)

- 1 whole-wheat or whole-grain bagel toasted
- 2 tbsp (28 g) light cream cheese
- 4 oz (113 g) smoked salmon
- 4 slices cucumbers
- 4 slices tomato
- 2 slices red onion
- 1 medium apple

Spread cream cheese onto bagel. Top with smoked salmon (lox), cucumber, tomato, and onion. Serve with an apple.

Carbohydrates: 38 g • Protein: 28 g • Fat: 14 g

Healthy Bacon and Eggs

- 3 large egg whites
- 2 oz (57 g) extra-lean Canadian style bacon
- 1½ tsp (7 ml) olive oil
- ½ grapefruit
- ¾ cup of blueberries

Spray a nonstick pan with an olive oil spray. Add egg whites and cook until set. Lightly coat another pan with oil. Prepare bacon following package instructions. Serve with a side of fruit.

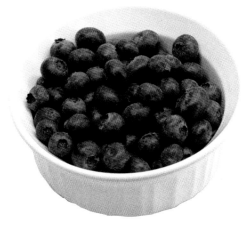

Carbohydrates: 30 g • Protein: 25 g • Fat: 10 g

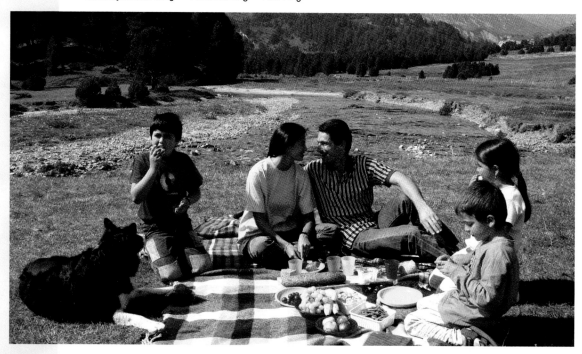

Ham and Swiss Crisp

- 3 slices Wasa fiber rye crispbread
- 3 oz (85 g) extra-lean sliced ham
- 1 oz (28 g) non-fat Swiss cheese
- 1 tsp (5 ml) mustard
- 1 tsp (5 ml) mayonnaise
- 1 leaf of loose-leaf lettuce

Spread mustard and mayonnaise on crisp bread. Top with ham, cheese, and lettuce. Enjoy with your choice of fruit on the side.

Carbohydrates: 38 g • Protein: 25 g • Fat: 11 g

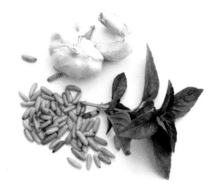

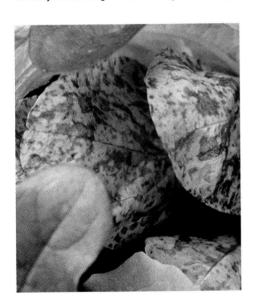

Pesto Tuna Melt

- 2 slices Wasa fiber crispbread or multi-grain bread
- 1 tbsp (15 ml) pesto sauce
- 3 oz (85 g) canned light tuna
- 1 oz (28 g) non-fat mozzarella cheese
- 2 slices tomato
- 1 serving fruit of choice

Spread pesto on crispbread. Top with tomato, tuna, and cheese. Put on foil in toaster oven or under broiler. Cook for a few minutes until cheese is melted. Serve with your choice of fruit for dessert.

Carbohydrates: 41 g • Protein: 37 g • Fat: 13 g

Deli Chicken Sandwich and Tossed Salad

- 2 slices multi-grain or whole-wheat bread
- 3 oz (85 g) chicken breast lunch meat
- 1 oz (28 g) low-fat Swiss cheese
- 1 tbsp (15 g) mustard
- 2 cups lettuce
- ½ cup (115 g) sliced cucumber
- 2 tomato slices
- 1 tbsp (15 g) fat-free Italian dressing
- 1 apple

Spread mustard onto toasted bread and top with cheese and sliced deli chicken. Serve with a side salad (lettuce, cucumber, tomato, and fat-free Italian dressing). Enjoy with an apple for dessert.

Carbohydrates: 41 g • Protein: 28 g • Fat: 11 g

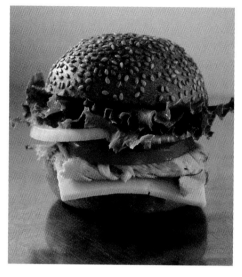

Tofu and Bean Salad

- 6 oz (170 g) light, extra-firm, silken tofu
- 1 cup canned dark red kidney beans
- 1 oz (28 g) sliced pitted green olives
- 2 tbsp (28 g) chopped parsley
- ½ tbsp (7 ml) extra-virgin olive oil
- ¼ tsp (1.2 ml) lemon juice
- Salt and pepper to taste

Mix all ingredients in a bowl. Chill and serve.

Carbohydrates: 45 g • Protein: 26 g • Fat: 13 g

Classic Turkey, Lettuce, and Tomato Sandwich

- 2 slices whole-wheat bread
- 2 tbsp (30 ml) Dijon mustard
- 3 slices roasted turkey breast
- 1 oz (28 g) low-fat cheese
- 2 slices tomato
- 1 apple

Spread Dijon mustard on bread. Top with turkey, cheese, lettuce, and tomato. Serve with an apple for dessert.

Carbohydrates: 43 g • Protein: 28 g • Fat: 13 g

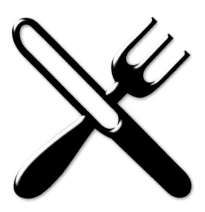

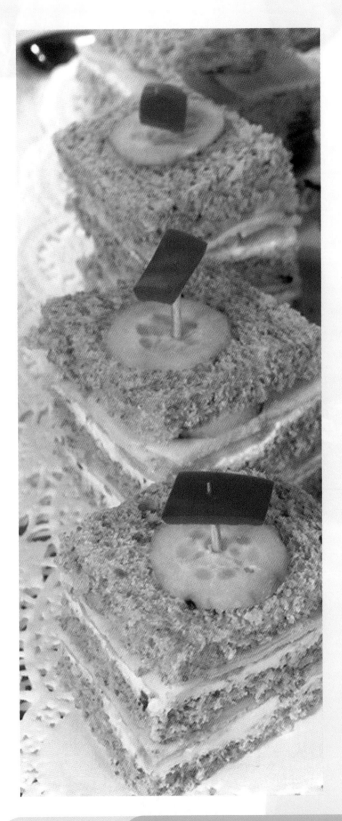

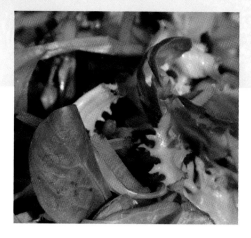

Speedy Sesame Tuna

- 3 oz (85 g) raw yellow fin tuna
- 1 tsp (5 ml) sesame oil
- 1 tsp (5 g) sesame seed
- 1 sweet potato baked with skin
- ³/₄ cup (172 g) boiled and chopped broccoli
- 2 cups lettuce
- ½ cup cucumber
- 2 slices tomato
- 1 tbsp (15 ml) balsamic vinegar
- 1 tsp (5 ml) extra-virgin olive oil

Preheat a pan or grill and add oil when hot. Season tuna with salt and pepper if desired. Add tuna to hot pan or grill and cook for 10 minutes, turning half way through, until tuna is cooked. Sprinkle with sesame seeds and cook for another minute. Serve with sweet potato, broccoli, and a tossed salad (lettuce, cucumber, tomato, balsamic vinegar, olive oil).

Carbohydrates: 44 g • Protein: 28 g • Fat: 11 g

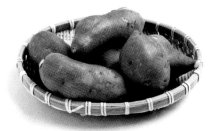

Grilled Chicken with Sweet Mandarin Salsa

- 4 oz (113 g) boneless and skinless chicken breast
- ½ cup (115 g) canned mandarin oranges
- 1 tbsp (15 ml) reserved mandarin juice
- ¼ cup (57 g) sliced red onion
- 2½ tsp (12 ml) extra-virgin olive oil
- 1 tbsp (15 ml) red wine vinegar
- 1 cup (230 g) broccoli florets
- 2 cups lettuce
- ½ cup sliced cucumber
- 2 tomato slices
- 1 tbsp (15 ml) balsamic vinegar
- 1 tbsp (15 ml) olive oil

In a bowl, mix mandarin oranges with reserved mandarin juice from can, onion, oil, vinegar, and salt and pepper to taste. Cover and refrigerate for a few hours. Grill chicken breast until chicken is no longer pink inside. Top with mandarin orange salsa. Serve with steamed broccoli and tossed salad (lettuce, cucumber, tomato, balsamic vinegar, olive oil).

Carbohydrates: 36 g • Protein: 28 g • Fat: 12 g

Log on to www.truestarhealth.com to create a personal nutritional meal plan based on your weight-loss goals, physical activity level, and current health status.

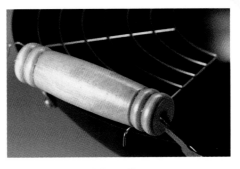

Tofu Chili

- 4 oz (113 g) light, extra-firm, silken tofu
- 4 oz (113 g) canned kidney beans
- ¼ cup (57 g)canned diced tomatoes
- ¾ cup (172 g) sliced mushrooms
- 2½ tsp (12 g) chopped onion
- 1½ tsp (7 ml) extra-virgin olive oil
- 1½ tsp (7 g) chili seasoning
- 1½ tsp (7 ml) tomato paste
- 2 oz (57 g) low-fat cheddar cheese

In a large pan, heat oil over medium-high heat and cook onion until soft. Crumble tofu into pan and add chili seasoning. Stir in tomato paste. Add remaining ingredients and simmer until thoroughly cooked, adding water as needed to create desired consistency. Serve with shredded cheese on top.

Carbohydrates: 41 g • Protein: 32 g • Fat: 12 g

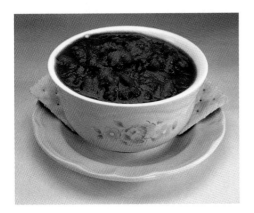

Cashew Beef Stir-Fry

- 2 tsp (10 ml) teriyaki sauce
- 1½ (tsp (7 ml) sesame oil
- ½ tsp (2.5 g) cornstarch
- 3½ oz (100 g) rib eye or round steak
- 1½ cup (345 g) sliced raw green pepper
- 1½ cup (345 g) sliced carrot
- ½ cup (115 g) chopped onion
- ¾ tsp (4 g) chopped cashews
- ½ cup (115 g) cubed cantaloupe

In a bowl, whisk together teriyaki sauce, ½ teaspoon of sesame oil, and corn-starch. Add beef strips and marinate in fridge for 30 minutes. Combine sauce, beef and vegetables in a wok and cook until meat is tender. Spoon onto a plate, sprinkle with cashews, and enjoy with ½ cup of cubed cantaloupe for dessert.

Carbohydrates: 39 g • Protein: 26 g • Fat: 12 g

Tasty Grilled Salmon

- 5 oz (141 g) salmon fillet (wild Atlantic if possible)
- 1 medium sweet potato
- 1 lemon
- lettuce
- tomato
- cucumber
- 1 tsp (15 ml) balsamic vinaigrette
- 1 tsp (15 ml) extra-virgin olive oil
- 1 tbsp (15 g) fresh dill

Preheat grill or oven to 375°F. Season salmon with lemon juice and dill sprigs. Cook on 375°F for 10-12 minutes. Bake or microwave sweet potato. Toss salad and enjoy!

Carbohydrates: 38 g • Protein: 30 g • Fat: 11 g

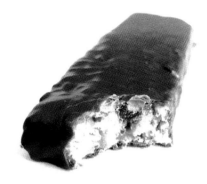

Snack Options

- Low-fat cheese with fruit
- Chick pea dip and veggies
- Strawberry banana smoothie with protein powder
- Soy nuts and fruit trail mix
- Protein bars
- Low-fat yogurt or cottage cheese with walnuts

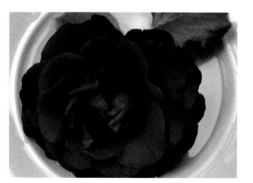

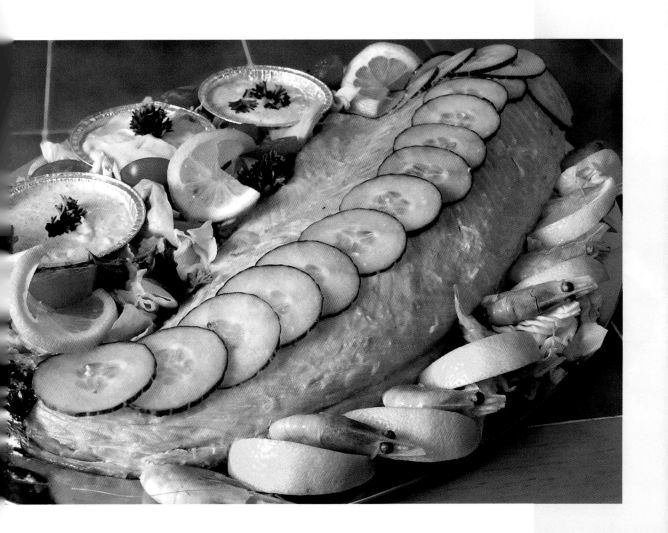

Corinne Zimperi

It didn't even feel like I was dieting!

How Truestar Way Changed My Life

Where do I possibly begin? Many years ago, I was an avid bodybuilder and prided myself on my looks. My husband was also a bodybuilder, and we enjoyed going to the gym together. I was also working as a constable for the city police force and my job required that I be in excellent physical shape.

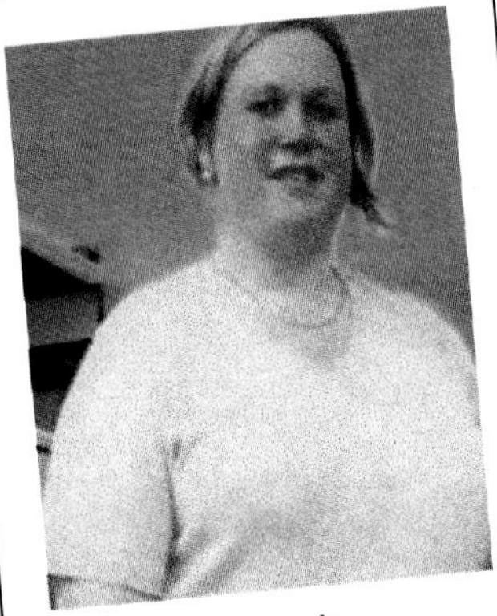

Before: 229 pounds

Then, everything changed in 1990 when I was diagnosed with cancer. I was put on hormone therapy and gradually began to gain weight. I was also experiencing low energy because of the treatments and stopped going to the gym. Before I knew it, it was 10 years later and I was 50 pounds heavier.

The past two years have been an emotional roller-coaster ride for me. I was laid off from my job and decided to go back to school to become a Social Worker and Drug and Alcohol Counselor. I was halfway through my first year of college when I experienced a devastating loss. I dropped in to visit my father and found him dead in his chair. To make matters worse, I couldn't take time off to recover because I had to complete exams.

I coped with all the stress in my life by turning to food for comfort.

With all of this trauma in my life, I was amazed to have achieved a 4.0 grade point average and to have received many awards of excellence. Going to school at this time was also difficult because I had an active 4-year-old at home. I coped with all the stress in my life by turning to food for comfort. I didn't have energy to play with my daughter Erika, my husband found me to be irritable all the time, and I continued to put on weight.

I knew I couldn't keep avoiding my weight-gain problems. I had to make changes in my life. A turning point came when my husband told me that if I couldn't lose weight for myself, I had to do it for my daughter because she deserved to have a mother around for many years. She needed a mother who

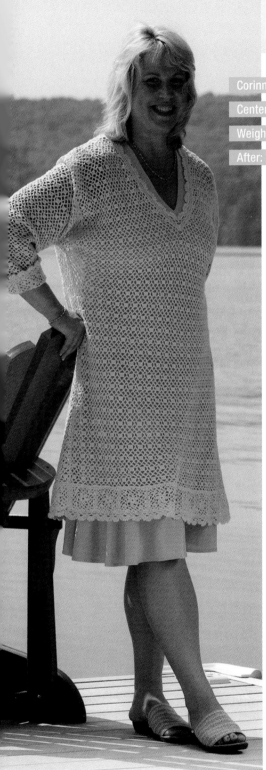

Corinne Zimperi

Center Location: Timmins

Weight Loss: 51 pounds / 39 inches

After: 178 pounds

had the energy to play with her — and he was right. I was only 40, but felt more like I was 80. My knees and back hurt, and I was in no shape to play with Erika.

Last Christmas, my husband gave me a life-changing present — a one-year membership to a Truestar for Women Nutrition & Fitness Centers. I joined Truestar on January 2 and my new year's resolution was to lose 40 pounds. Well, thanks to the Truestar program and its wonderful team of professionals, I am close to realizing my weight-loss goal. The nutritional program is easy to follow and to incorporate in my family meals. I loved the diet program. It didn't even feel like I was dieting! Truestar introduced me to a variety of foods, and the supplements gave me the extra energy I needed to help me reach my weight-loss goal. I have 3 more pounds to go until I hit my goal. And, even better, I have the energy to try bodybuilding again!

Thank you, Truestar! My 6-year-old daughter Erika also says, "Thank you, Truestar, for helping my mommy to lose weight. She now plays hopscotch and skipping with me and takes me to the park, too."

Thanks to the Truestar program and its wonderful team of professionals, I am close to realizing my weight-loss goal.

Exercise

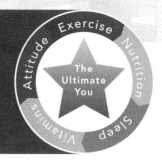

The Ultimate You

Attitude · Exercise · Nutrition · Sleep · Vitamins

Let There Be "Exercise" in Your Day!

Tim Mulcahy

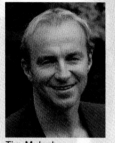

Tim Mulcahy

Once I became involved in the sales world, I adopted the customary health regimen of its 'players' — a diet of fast food at McDonald's or Burger King, lots of coffee, and a half-pack of cigarettes a day.

When I was 16, I left home and began selling vacuum cleaners for Filter Queen Vacuum. Until then, I had been fairly active in sports, playing high-school basketball and competitive baseball and hockey, with some track and field thrown in. Even as a child, my habit had been to be out in the world, mobile and curious. Once I became involved in the sales world, however, I adopted the customary health regimen of its 'players' — a diet of fast food at McDonald's or Burger King, lots of coffee, and a half-pack of cigarettes a day. As my consumption of empty carbs, sugar and, nicotine went up, my active lifestyle went down (the drain), unless you include hitting the odd disco on a Friday or Saturday night as a form of exercise. I was on a collision course with poor health.

At the time, I simply wasn't aware of what I was doing to my health, but I did sense that I was doing something to my daily energy level and ability to focus. To me, that was an even more serious issue. I soon graduated from selling vacuum cleaners to home insulation. The year was 1982 and I was 20 years old. Despite my poor lifestyle choices, my sales career had continued to improve. I was in commission-based, door-to-door sales and one of the key components to being a good salesman in an industry where most fail is your energy level. I always had a fairly positive attitude and derived my energy from my attitude (certainly not from my diet and exercise regimen).

One day I was asked by my employer to field-train two new sales agents, Derek Goodman and Mike Edgson. When I first met them for lunch at Swiss Chalet, they were already eating their chicken, but oddly enough, they had removed the skin. "Why are you taking off the best part," I asked them. They looked at each other and rolled their eyes. Derek looked like The Incredible Hulk, and Mike, like The Hulk's younger brother. They had owned a gym

> "A woman's health can be judged by which she takes two at a time — pills or stairs."
> Joan Welsh

together that had just gone under, and that's why they had taken the job selling home insulation door to door. Derek Goodman had been a former Mr Eastern Canada, and Mike had been a fitness instructor with Vic Tanny's health club before going into business for himself.

When I told them that selling insulation was easier in smaller communities, Mike proposed we work out of his in-law's farm in Coldwater, a farming and cottage community about an hour north of Toronto. The first morning when we awoke Mike suggested we go for a run, something I hadn't done for at least 4 years. We ran down to the stop sign and back, about 2 miles. I was having trouble keeping up, but I didn't want to give up. I hate quitting, but when I finished the run, I felt ill and had to fight back nausea for several minutes.

Then it happened. After having a shower and starting to get dressed, I noticed that my eyes were glowing — in fact, my whole face was glowing. My cheeks were ruddy and I felt great. The endorphins had kicked in, something I hadn't felt in over 4 years, and I was on a high. It didn't stop there.

The next day Mike suggested we lift some weights. I was game. When we went outside to the bench press, Mike suggested I warm up with 80 lbs. "Sure thing," I said, but ended up needing a spot because my muscle development had been almost non-existent since the age of 16. A few days later, he suggested

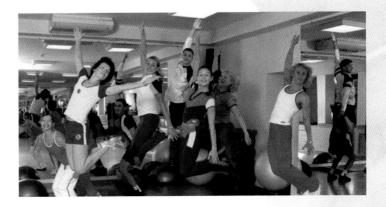

tennis, and after that I was hooked.

Before work each day, we would run or play tennis or pump some iron. The direct outcome — my sales increased. My focus was greater, my body language was better as my posture and physique had improved, and I had more confidence. In the following year, my personal income jumped 100%. There was no doubt in my mind that it was mainly due to the way my new regular exercise routine had begun to restore balance to my very unbalanced life.

Throughout the years I've continued to work out. Today, I exercise 6 days a week on average (prior to work on weekdays) and alternate cardio and weight training. I don't know how I would be able to remain focused without my daily workout regimen, because every day I exercise, I feel better than any day I don't. I feel healthier and more energized.

Oh yes, the indirect outcome of my exercise program — exercise became the second principle of the Truestar way to lifelong health and wellness.

> Then it happened. After having a shower and starting to get dressed, I noticed that my eyes were glowing — in fact, my whole face was glowing.

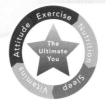

Exercise the Truestar Way

Michael Carrera, M.Sc.
Vice-President, Exercise Planning & Development

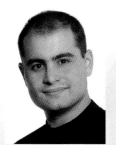

Michael Carrera

Clearly, the better your level of fitness, the lower your risk of disease and death. Knowing this, then why aren't we more active?

Exercise is a cornerstone of good health, one of the five principles of the Truestar way — nutrition, exercise, vitamins, attitude, and sleep. Despite the solid scientific information available regarding the benefits of regular exercise, nearly 60% of North American adults are not regularly active and, surprisingly, 25% are not active at all. These stats also help explain why approximately two-thirds of our population is overweight and one-third obese.

Excusitis

From time to time, many of us suffer from 'excusitis'. We know what we need to do, but we find a way of sabotaging our best intentions. "I am too tired," we say to excuse ourselves from exercising. "I have to cook dinner," we plead. "The

HEALTH RISKS

Let's take a look at some of the health risks of not exercising regularly. The facts are startling.

☐ **Cardiovascular Risk**
Low levels of physical activity are associated with an increased risk of cardiovascular disease. Many long-term studies on both men and women have reported a 30% to 50% increase in the risk of developing high blood pressure due to an inactive lifestyle.

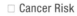

☐ **Cancer Risk**
Regular physical exercise protects against developing many site-specific cancers, including breast, prostate, colon, and rectal cancer. The protective effect of exercise can be as high as 50%.

☐ **Death Risk**
People who are sedentary are two times more likely to die prematurely than people who regularly exercise and keep fit.

Clearly, the better your level of fitness, the lower your risk of disease and death. Knowing this, then why aren't we more active?

kids take up so much of my time." Once we get beyond these daily living excuses, we find the 'professional' excuse handy. "There are so many experts on fitness with so many different programs that I just don't know where to start."

No more excuses! Start today and exercise following the program in the next few pages or by using the enclosed Truestar Workout DVD. You can exercise in the comfort of your own home.

Exercise Myths

Excusitis is not the only barrier to exercising daily. Some people have false notions about the kind of exercise that is best for weight loss and optimal health. These myths get in the way of developing an effective and safe exercise program. Let's dispel them here at the outset so we aren't troubled by them further.

MYTH #1:

Fat-Burning Zone

Quite often you hear people talking about exercising in their "fat-burning zone." The fat-burning zone was first popularized during the early 1990's fitness craze when the 'no pain/no gain' approach was replaced by low-intensity exercise as the way to lose weight. Unfortunately, people have taken this term to heart, believing that exercising in this low-intensity zone actually burns a greater amount of fat.

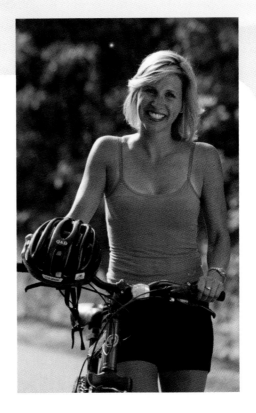

Reality

Here is how you maximize your fat-burning potential. If intensity was rated on a scale of 1 to 10, with 10 being extremely difficult, you should focus your energy on achieving a 7 or 8, and occasionally going for a 9.

Exercising with a heart rate value equivalent to 65% to 85% of your maximum heart rate is comfortable and manageable, providing the greatest calorie burn when you are performing a circuit or cardiovascular activity. On average, most people only exercise for 20 to 30 minutes consecutively.

Wouldn't it be best to optimize your calorie-burning potential! When performing your circuit-training workout, focus on pushing yourself to a limit you feel you can comfortably maintain.

Here is how you maximize your fat burning potential. If intensity was rated on a scale of 1 to 10, with 10 being extremely difficult, you should focus your energy on achieving a 7 or 8 and occasionally going for a 9.

MYTH #2:

Spot Reduction and Spot Toning

The idea that if you want to lose fat around the mid-section, hips, or thighs, all you have to do is exercise that area and the fat will 'melt away' is a myth. When you perform physical activity, either structured (such as circuit training) or unstructured (such as grocery shopping or mowing the lawn), your body mobilizes and burns fat from your *entire* body. Your body does not discriminate when it comes to fat loss. There are some minor differences between men and woman. In general, men will lose weight in the lower body, followed by the arms and abdomen. Women will lose the weight in their abdomen first, then in their arms, and finally in their lower body.

Reality

While there is no such thing as spot reduction, you can 'spot tone'. In order to tone a muscle, you must work a muscle. You cannot tighten your thighs by strength training your arms. Muscle toning is site specific and requires the use of resistance in order to stimulate lean muscle growth. Multi-joint exercises are great because they work more than one muscle group at a time. For example, a dumbbell bicep curl is a single joint exercise, while the dumbbell squat is a multi-joint exercise.

So, spot reduction is possible as long as the goal is to spot reduce throughout the entire body. Spot toning is site specific and can be achieved by strictly focusing on the muscle group you wish to tone. Be patient and consistent and the results will follow.

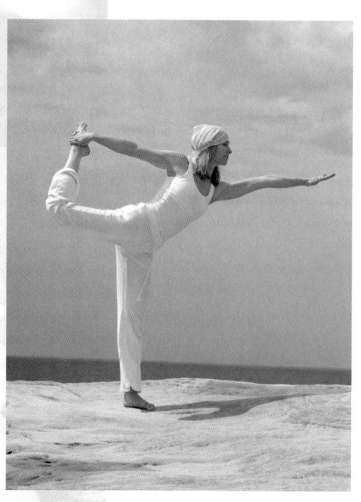

FITNESS EQUATION:

$$\text{Overall Reduction} + \text{Spot Toning} = \text{The Ultimate You}$$

Log on to www.truestarhealth.com to create a personal exercise plan based on your weight-loss goals, physical activity level, and current health status.

MYTH #3:

Muscle Weighs More than Fat

That muscle weighs more than fat is a common myth in fitness circles, but what weighs more — 10 pounds of lead or 10 pounds of feathers, as the old saying goes? I love to watch the expression of Truestar members during our seminars when we dispel this myth!

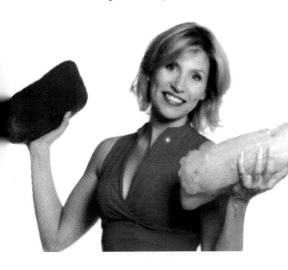

Reality

Muscle does not weigh more than fat. Ten pounds of muscle weigh the same as 10 pounds of fat. The misunderstanding comes from the fact that the same amount of muscle has less volume than the same weight in fat. In other words, 10 pounds of muscle is denser and actually looks smaller than 10 pounds of fat. It is also true that muscle is metabolically active, so that the more muscle you have, the greater the number of calories you burn at rest.

SCENARIO 1

If you have very little weight to lose (for example, 3 to 15 pounds), you may think that your resistance-training program is not helping you lose weight. You may actually gain a few pounds, but look slimmer, have greater tone, and lose inches. This is why when you want to lose very little weight, it's not a good idea to use the scale as a guide or reference point. You may weigh more but take up less room. Your body has, in fact, become denser. This is the reason we rely on measuring inches of weight loss rather than simply relying on the scale.

SCENARIO 2

If you want to lose a higher amount of weight (15 to 30+ pounds), you will gain muscle, lose body fat, and lose weight on the scale. Research on young athletes has shown that every person gains muscle in different amounts over a certain amount of time. The maximum amount of muscle that a human being can probably gain in a year is 25 pounds of lean muscle mass. The focus of the Truestar exercise program is not to stimulate large amounts of muscle growth, but rather an increase in metabolism by promoting muscle tone, fat loss, and lean muscle growth. Since the gain in muscle is not as fast as the total weight lost (both fat and water), a person who needs to lose a relatively higher amount of weight will reduce body fat, gain lean muscle mass, and reduce total body weight, simultaneously.

Muscle is metabolically active, so that the more muscle you have, the greater the number of calories you burn at rest.

The focus of the Truestar exercise program is not to stimulate large amounts of muscle growth, but rather an increase in metabolism by promoting muscle tone, fat loss, and lean muscle growth.

MYTH # 4:

Cardiovascular Exercise Is Best for Fat Loss

A single session of 30 minutes of cardiovascular activity will burn substantially more calories than 30 minutes of resistance training. For this reason, it is falsely believed that cardiovascular exercise is best for fat loss.

Reality

In fact, fat loss is best achieved with a proper combination of cardiovascular and strength training, combined with better eating habits and vitamin supplements. In order to lose 1 pound of fat, you must expend 3500 calories. In other words, to lose 1 pound of fat per week, you have to create a calorie deficit of at least 500 calories per day for 7 days. This caloric deficit can be created by following the Truestar way of eating, taking supplements, and increasing daily exercise or energy expenditure.

When you burn calories during a cardiovascular session, your metabolism increases for a very short period of time. While strength training burns fewer calories per session, you burn more calories throughout the day — yes, even while you sleep — as a direct consequence of building muscle. It is estimated that 1 pound of muscle burns approximately 35 to 50 extra calories per day. If you gain 10 pounds of muscle over the course of a year, you burn an extra 350 to 500 calories per day and an extra 2450 to 3500 calories per week just by engaging in regular short bursts of resistance training. Combining strength training with cardiovascular training in a circuit-training program is the fastest and most efficient method of fat loss.

> Fat loss is best achieved with a proper combination of cardiovascular and strength training, combined with better eating habits and vitamin supplements.

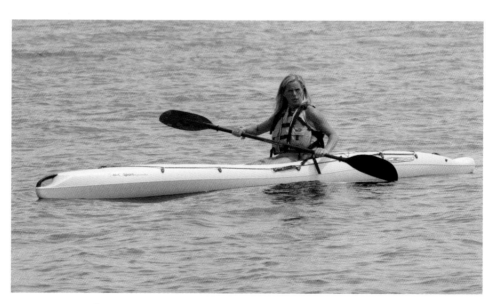

MYTH # 5:

You Gain Muscle while You Exercise

Some people believe that you gain muscle strength and growth during exercise. The harder and more frequently you exercise, the more your muscles grow. This is not only false, but potentially dangerous.

Reality

We have all heard the saying "less is more." Well, this also applies to exercise. Our muscles heal and grow for 24 to 48 hours *after* the workout session, not during the session. When a muscle is inflicted with the stress of a workout session, it undergoes a process known as the General Adaptation Syndrome (GAS). When the muscle is 'broken down' by the workout, the body provides nutrients to enable the muscle to heal, repair, and grow. In time, usually 24 to 48 hours, the muscle adapts, becoming stronger and wiser than it was prior to the workout session. However, if a second resistance training session occurs before the muscles can heal and grow, your results will be halted and your progress stunted.

This is why it is important to perform a strength-training program every other day or at least alternate the muscle groups you exercise if you train 2 days in a row. In order to gain muscle, you need to strength train two to four times a week. Three times a week is ideal. As for

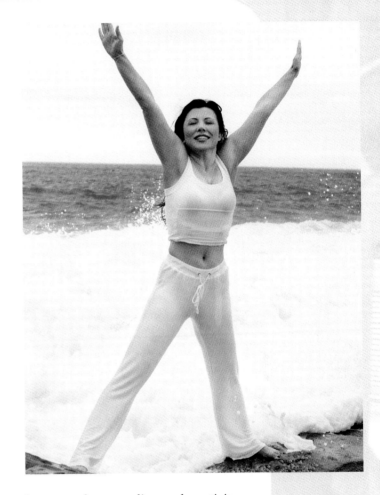

low to moderate cardiovascular activity, our bodies replenish their energy stores quite quickly, so cardiovascular sessions can be performed on a daily basis.

Be careful and make sure you give your body adequate time to rest and recover. Listen to your body — it will let you know when it needs a day off from training. To help it heal, get plenty of sleep, eat highly nutritious foods, and take any necessary vitamin supplements required for optimum health.

Make sure you give your body adequate time to rest and recover.

Getting Started

We will guide you every step of the Truestar way to becoming the Ultimate You by achieving your weight loss, health, and fitness goals.

Well, put the excuses and myths aside and let's get started. We are not asking for much, just a minimum of 30 minutes, three times per week, on alternate days. If you are able to participate in some extra cardiovascular exercise during the week, such as going for a walk or bike ride, great! If not, that's okay, too, as long as you follow the Truestar program three times a week. If you want to exercise more often, that's fine, too.

We've made the program simple to follow so you don't have to think hard about it or get confused with complex terms and procedures. You don't have to worry about counting reps or how long to rest between sets. The program does not require elaborate or expensive equipment. You can make do with household items. We've also included photos and a description of exercises that you can perform anywhere and anytime. The program even comes with a unique workout DVD that you can watch in the comfort of your own home. We will guide you every step of the Truestar way to becoming the Ultimate You by achieving your weight loss, health, and fitness goals.

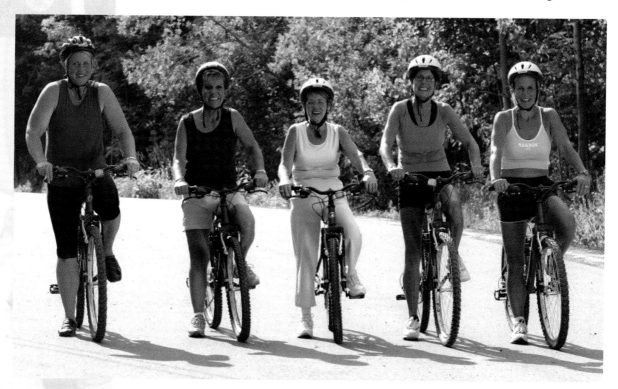

truestarhealth.com

Log on to www.truestarhealth.com to create a personal exercise plan based on your weight-loss goals, physical activity level, and current health status.

Three Kinds of Exercise

1. Strength Training

These exercises are designed to increase muscle strength and endurance. Muscle strength is your ability to contract a muscle against resistance, such as weights, stationary equipment, or body weight. Muscle endurance is your ability to contract a muscle repeatedly. In other words, muscle strength is how much you can lift (or resist) and muscle endurance is how long you can lift for (or resist). For this reason, strength training is often called resistance training. Strength-training exercises are typically repeated a number of times. These repetitions or 'reps' are usually part of a 'set' of exercises. In general, exercises to improve muscle strength involve sets with higher resistance and a lower number of reps, while exercises to increase muscle endurance involve sets with lower resistance and a higher number of reps.

2. Cardiovascular Training

These exercises are designed to increase lung capacity and heart rate, causing blood to circulate more efficiently around the body and to deliver more oxygen to the muscles. Sometimes called aerobics, 'cardio' exercises improve overall health and expend energy stored as fat in the body. Walking, jogging, running, and

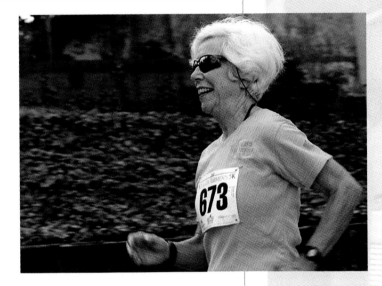

swimming, as well as working out on a treadmill or elliptical machine, are common forms of cardio exercise. Cardio exercises are measured by their frequency, duration, and intensity.

3. Circuit Training

Circuit-training programs, similar to the exercises on the enclosed Truestar Workout DVD, combine strength exercises and cardiovascular exercises conducted relatively quickly at a series of 'stations' for short periods of time. Going quickly from one exercise station to another keeps the heart rate elevated in the calorie-burning zone and promotes overall fitness by working all muscle groups, as well as the heart and the lungs.

Principles of the Truestar Exercise Program

The best way to avoids myths and live in the "real" world is by following principles built on a solid scientific foundation. That's the Truestar way of developing a safe and effective exercise program.

1. Combine Strength and Cardio Exercise in a Circuit Training Program

My work designing high-performance exercise programs for athletes has taught me the benefits of using strength and cardiovascular exercise phases in a circuit-training fashion.

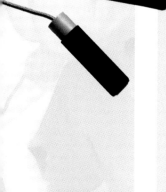

That is the beauty of the Truestar program — a higher level of fitness achieved in less time.

CIRCUIT TRAINING BENEFITS

- ☐ Increased strength and muscular endurance
- ☐ Increased lean muscle mass (which increases metabolism)
- ☐ Improved blood sugar levels and insulin response
- ☐ Improved immunity
- ☐ Improved bone health
- ☐ Improved blood pressure, cholesterol levels, and heart function
- ☐ Improved cardiovascular fitness
- ☐ Improvement in psychological health
- ☐ Improved self-esteem and self-confidence
- ☐ Improved attitude
- ☐ Improved sleep
- ☐ Climbing stairs will never seem so easy

In this way, our bodies are constantly challenged with new exercises or different ways of performing an exercise. In turn, circuit training stimulates greater results in the same amount of workout time. That is the beauty of the Truestar program — a higher level of fitness achieved in less time. To top it off, our circuit-training program is based on good science so we don't jeopardize your health. Indeed, the Truestar circuit-training program enhances your overall health.

Scientific studies have investigated the relative effect of following a strength-training program, a cardiovascular-training program, or a circuit-training program on metabolism, body fat, muscle strength, and cardiovascular fitness. The results prove the superior value of circuit training.

Strength training and cardiovascular training offer different benefits that are combined in circuit training. Strength training shapes and tones your body and revs-up your metabolism by increasing your lean muscle mass. Cardiovascular training within approximately 65% to 85% of your maximum heart rate range improves the efficiency of heart and lungs and burns many calories. Sequencing strength training with cardiovascular training in a timed circuit not only combines their benefits but can enhance the benefits of both

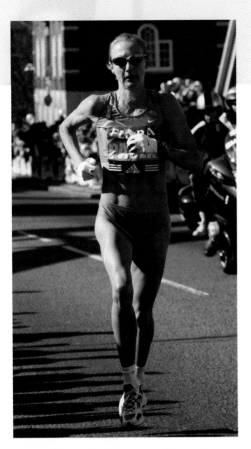

types of exercise. For example, moving from one strength-training exercise to the next non-stop in a circuit burns approximately 25% more calories than resistance training alone.

Circuit training is the best training method for building muscle strength, reducing body fat, increasing metabolism, and improving cardiovascular fitness. Circuit training also has a positive effect on our sense of well-being or attitude, another Truestar principle of good health. A recent study of a 6-week circuit-training program followed by college students showed significant improvements in their self-evaluation of their physical appearance and body composition, with reduced social anxiety and enhanced physical self-efficacy.

2. Follow a Proper Progression

There are many ways to progress through an exercise program. With resistance training, you can change the weight, the reps, the sets, or rest intervals between sets. With cardio training, you can train at a higher heart rate range for a longer period of time or use interval training, alternating a more intense activity, such as sprinting on a treadmill for 2 minutes, with 5 minutes of lower intensity activity, such as jogging or walking.

We have designed a natural progression of exercises in three phases — beginner, intermediate, and advanced. You can individualize your circuit, mixing and matching exercises from each phase, and progress from one phase to the next at your own rate. You don't have to worry about what comes next. We don't even use reps or rest intervals between sets. Just follow the program at your own pace and comfort level.

3. Add Spice

Variety is the spice of life — and spice will keep you motivated to exercise. Trying new routines that exercise new muscles or the same muscles in new ways keeps the program fun and the results enduring. Our bodies are very plastic and love to adapt to new and exciting experiences. Variety in the Truestar workout is achieved by alternating exercises and by challenging the body to push harder by using a phase-based training approach. At Truestarhealth.com, you will find over

Sequencing strength training with cardiovascular training in a timed circuit not only combines their benefits but can enhance the benefits of both types of exercise.

We have designed a natural progression of exercises in three phases —beginner, intermediate, and advanced. You can individualize your circuit, mixing and matching exercises from each phase, and progress from one phase to the next at your own rate.

Just three times a week. No long waits for exercise machines. No complicated instructions. And only 30 minutes. It's that simple.

Even one full round of the circuit can help you maintain your level of fitness and keep you motivated.

3,000 exercise videos — a wealth of spices. If you ever need a change in routine, you are one or two clicks away from learning a new exercise to tighten your glutes or strengthen your abs!

4. Simplify, Simplify

In a maximum of 30 minutes, you can properly warm-up, complete an exhilarating and energizing exercise circuit, and cool-down to prepare to tackle the rest of the day. In just half an hour, you can perform a safe and effective circuit-training routine, in your home, that combines exercises targeting the entire body. Each of the exercise stations includes "recovery time," which allows you to exercise at your own pace and in your own way. During the recovery period, simply walk on the spot and stretch the muscle group you just finished working. Relax and prepare your body for the next station. If you are advanced, simply move from one station to the next non-stop.

Just three times a week. No long waits for exercise machines. No complicated instructions. And only 30 minutes. It's that simple.

5. Use It or Lose It

The principle of reversibility simply states that if you don't use it, you will lose it. The gains you fought so hard to achieve will quickly be lost if you stop exercising. Your metabolism will return to pre-exercise levels, your gains in

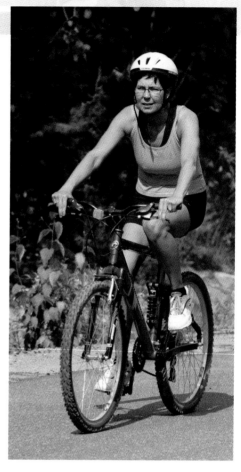

strength and endurance will diminish, and, even if you don't deviate from your nutrition plan, you may find yourself regaining some of the weight you lost.

As a rule of thumb, if you must cut back on the frequency of workouts, bump up the intensity. Exercise as hard as you can 1 to 2 days a week, and, if possible, complete a short 12-minute circuit (one full set of all the exercises) on another day. Even one full round of the circuit can help you maintain your level of fitness and keep you motivated. You have worked so hard to gain it, try not to lose it.

Log on to www.truestarhealth.com to create a personal exercise plan based on your weight-loss goals, physical activity level, and current health status.

6. Warm-up and Cool-Down

An improper warm-up is the main cause for injuries that occur during strength and cardiovascular training. We recommend performing some light calisthenic exercises, such as jogging on the spot for 2 to 3 minutes, and some light stretching before beginning the circuit. A warm muscle responds better to exercise than a cold muscle. After your workout is complete, take 2 to 3 minutes to perform the same stretches as you did warming up. This will give your body an opportunity to relax before resuming your daily activities and stretch the energized muscles back to their resting length. Perform 3 to 5 stretches and hold each stretch for 15 to 25 seconds.

7. Overcome Fatigue with Exercise Order

Eventually, fatigue will catch up to you regardless of what tactics you use to overcome it. Properly planning the order in which exercises are performed is a logical way of preventing or, at least, delaying the onset of fatigue. For instance, performing three upper body exercises in a row may be good for fitness, but will inevitably hamper your performance on subsequent exercises. Ideally, you would exercise the large muscle groups first, followed by the small muscle groups. By viewing the Truestar Workout DVD and visiting truestarhealth.com, you can discover a wealth of exercises. Alternate different exercises on different days and also in different orders, so that your body is always kept guessing and improving while providing the variety and excitement you need to keep moving.

8. Increase Reps First and Weight Second

This is a very important exercise principle. We want to make sure that you maximize the results you can achieve at every phase in your exercise program. If you begin to exercise at 30-second intervals as a beginner at a moderate pace, you should first increase the time you perform each exercise by moving onto the 45-second and 60-second interval before increasing the weight you use. This will insure proper progression, maximize your muscle endurance potential, and improve your fitness. Oh yeah, it helps you burn more calories too!

> Properly planning the order in which exercises are performed is a logical way of preventing or, at least, delaying the onset of fatigue.

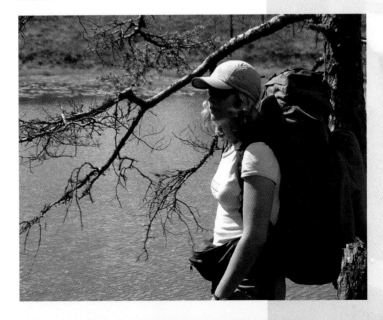

Truestar Exercise Program

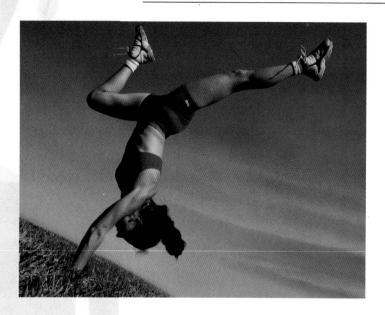

You'll soon begin to look forward each week to these sessions. They will become a special time just for you.

Start the exercises on the Truestar Workout DVD today.

Program Phases

The program is staged in three phases of training conducted at progressively higher levels of intensity, geared for beginner (Phase I), intermediate (Phase II), and advanced (Phase III) levels of experience and fitness.

For example, Phase I requires 30 seconds of non-stop resistance training, followed by 30 seconds of walking on the spot. Phase II places more emphasis on resistance training (45 seconds) and less on recovery (15 seconds). Phase III has you completing the workout non-stop for 60 seconds per station, as you move from one exercise to another.

Duration

The program has been designed to accommodate not only a 24-minute workout (excluding warm-up and cool-down) but also a 12-minute workout, by simply performing 1 set through the circuit instead of 2. Remember, variety is what ignites progress.

Following a program of this nature allows you to use resistance training for strength benefits, and the low impact non-stop activity keeps your heart rate

Program Stations

The Truestar exercise program consists of 12 stations per circuit for a total of 24 active minutes. Each station allows a maximum time of 60 seconds. That leaves 3 minutes for warm-up and 3 minutes for cool-down. Total time: 30 minutes.

Repeat each exercise on the circuit:
- ☐ 6 resistance training stations
- ☐ 3 core (abdominal/lower back) stations
- ☐ 3 specific cardio stations

PHASE	LEVEL	RESISTANCE EXERCISE TIME	RECOVERY TIME
I	Beginner	30 seconds	30 seconds
II	Intermediate	45 seconds	15 seconds
III	Advanced	60 seconds	0 seconds

elevated in what we like to call the optimal "calorie-burning" zone. Performing resistance training exercises non-stop will burn 25% more calories than resistance training with rest breaks in between exercises, elevating your metabolism for 24 to 48 hours after your exercise session. Now, that's progress!

Rhythm

Perform your circuit-training workout a minimum of two to three times a week, preferably on alternate days. For instance, depending on your schedule, you may exercise first thing in the morning on Monday, again on Wednesday, and then after work on Friday. Try to get into a regular exercise rhythm or routine. You'll soon begin to look forward each week to these sessions. They will become a special time just for you.

Balance

Cardiovascular training is as important as resistance training, but traditionally cardio was believed to be the superior workout for burning fat. However, too much cardio can lead to a steady rise in a variety of stress hormones and can hurt your fat loss goals. The key is to follow a balanced approach.

We suggest performing a maximum of 1.5 to 2 hours of cardio per week in addition to your circuit-training program. On your off days from the circuit workout, go for a 30-minute walk, ride your bike, or jump on an elliptical machine. You don't have to perform all 30 minutes

MAXIMUM HEART RATE

To calculate your maximum heart rate range, use this formula: deduct your current age from 220 to arrive at your 'age-predicted maximum heart rate' (MHR), and then multiply this number by 65% and 85% to arrive at your 'heart rate range'.

☐ For example, let's say you are 30 years old:
220 – 30 (age) = 190 MHR
190 x 65% = 123
190 x 85% = 161

Therefore, the lower end of your heart rate range is 123 beats per minute and the higher range is 161. Attempt to keep your longer heart rate toward the higher end for a part of your cardio workout.

TALK TEST

If heart rate isn't something you like to use to gauge how hard you are working, then you can use something called the *Talk Test*. Increase your exercise intensity to the point where conversation is difficult, but not impossible.

at once, but should aim at having your heart rate within 65% to 85% of your 'age-predicted maximum heart rate' range for the duration of the workout.

Intervals

If you really want to rev-up your cardio workout, then go full throttle, but be cautious. Our bodies adapt quickly to the motor skill of riding a bike, walking on a treadmill, or exercising on an elliptical machine. Increasing the intensity by strictly raising the resistance works well for some people, but this can hinder the progress of others. If the resistance is too

Aim at having your heart rate within 65% to 85% of your 'age-predicted maximum heart rate' range for the duration of the workout.

high, fatigue can set in prematurely, which doesn't help the already over-worked leg muscles.

Instead of performing continuous intense cardio, try interval training as an effective alternative. For instance, if you routinely exercise between levels 5 and 6 on the bike or elliptical trainer or walk at a certain pace, bump up the level for 2-minute segments. Either pedal faster at the same level of difficulty or increase the difficulty by 2 or 3 levels and pedal against a higher resistance. If walking, walk at a faster pace, jog, or walk up hill if you have that option. Either way, just

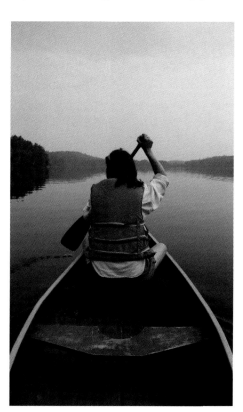

make the exercise more difficult for 2 minutes. Afterwards, decrease the resistance or speed to comfort level and recuperate for 5 minutes before starting the process again. Do this for the duration of your cardio workout.

Pace

The Truestar exercise program is not always easy, but the good news is that you can exercise at your own pace. Whether you are a beginner or experienced exerciser, we always suggest you start at Phase I of the exercise program. When you feel ready to move up to the next level, the transition is very easy. True beginners can perform each exercise with their body weight alone until they feel strong enough to attempt the exercises with a few small dumbbells. A true beginner workout is demonstrated in the Truestar Workout DVD.

When Phase I seems very easy, go to phase II and progress accordingly. Increase the time spent at each station before increasing the weight you use. This will guarantee that your body properly and efficiently adapts to the exercise program and that your level of conditioning will continue to increase.

Progress

You don't have to progress from a beginner to an intermediate exerciser overnight. Take your time. It can be a slow process. If you want to try an intermediate program, attempt a few exercises before just diving in with your entire

Instead of performing continuous intense cardio, try interval training as an effective alternative.

Increase the time spent at each station before increasing the weight you use.

You don't have to progress from a beginner to an intermediate exerciser overnight. Take your time.

Log on to www.truestarhealth.com to create a personal exercise plan based on your weight-loss goals, physical activity level, and current health status.

workout. For instance, of the 12 stations you perform, you may wish to perform the first 6 as a beginner and the next 6 as an intermediate, adding a new exercise at every workout until your entire program is intermediate. As an alternative, since you are completing 2 sets of the circuit, you can perform the first set as a beginner and the second set as an intermediate. It is totally up to you!

My Truestar 30-Minute Exercise Program

Here's what my daily exercise program looks like. I'm not an exercise fanatic by any means, but I look forward to my daily 30-minute workout sessions. This is what my schedule allows first thing in the morning, my best time to exercise. While I don't always have the most energy in the morning, my day just isn't the same if I don't get my workouts in. I set my schedule by one rule of thumb: *I feel better on the days I exercise than on the days I don't exercise.* Chances are this may also apply to you.

Sometimes I only perform a circuit-training workout and other times I finish my circuit training routine with 10 to 15 minutes of additional cardio. You may also have noticed that I don't always exercise at the same level. That is the beauty of the program; its *simplicity* allows you to individualize it and adapt it to how you are feeling.

Since Monday is usually a physically tough day for me, I prefer to start the week at Phase I. By the middle and end of the week, I am ready to tackle Phase II and sometimes aspire to Phase III. By the way, I generally try to take Saturday and Sunday off from formal exercise. I like to get outdoors and enjoy being active in nature. I recommend you do the same.

So, your program can look something like this, or you can modify it your way, or simply perform the basic circuit three times a week. Start slowly at a low to medium pace. Your goal should be to exercise for an entire phase without stopping. If you feel the need to stop, that's okay — just continue when you are ready. Judge how you feel at the end of the workout, not after a particular exercise. Moving up too fast can get you tired too quickly.

MONDAY	TUESDAY	WEDNESDAY	THURSDAY	FRIDAY
Circuit Training Phase I followed by 15 minutes of extra cardio	Cardio Training Exercise bike for 30 minutes at 65% to 85% MHR	Circuit Training Phase II No cardio	Cardio Training Exercise bike for 15 minutes, followed by 15 minutes on elliptical trainer at 65% to 85% MHR	Circuit Training Phase III No cardio

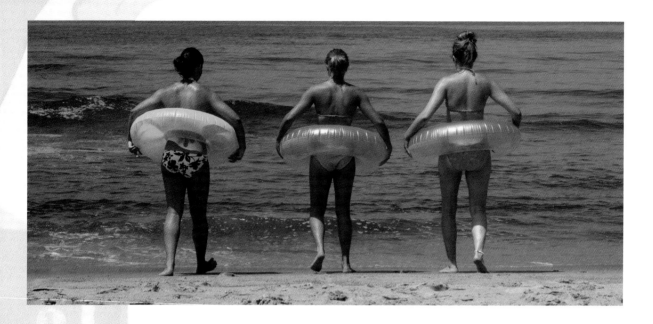

EQUIPMENT

For equipment, you can start with a simple pair of dumbbells, a bench, a cardio 'machine', your own body weight, and the Truestar Workout DVD.

☐ **Dumbbells:** Women can start with a dumbbell set of 5 LBS or 8 LBS and men with a set of 15 LBS or 20 LBS. Before you increase the weight, make sure you can complete the exercises for Phase III (60 seconds). When you do increase the weight, start at Phase I (30 seconds) and slowly progress toward Phase III.

☐ **Bench:** A flat to incline bench is handy, but not required. Most exercises can be performed without a bench. Log on at truestarhealth.com for alternative exercises that don't require this piece of equipment.

☐ **Cardio Machine:** You don't need to buy a cardio machine — just use what your environment offers. Walking outside, climbing stairs, riding your bike, swimming in the lake, or going for a jog are all good 'machines'.

☐ **Body Weight:** Body-weight exercises are ideal for improving your strength, so you will need your body, too! Login in at truestarhealth.com for more exercises using your body weight for resistance.

Truestar 30-Minute Exercise Program

Here is a quick reference chart for you to use in developing your own 30-minute program with 12 stations of exercise. Remember to start with a 3-minute warm-up and end with a 3-minute cool-down. For instructions on how to do each exercise, along with photos to help you see good form, follow this chart.

STATION #	EXERCISE/ STATION	PHASE I (Seconds)		PHASE II (Seconds)		PHASE III (Seconds)
1	Dumbbell Squat	30 active exercise	30 recovery time	45 active exercise	15 recovery time	60 active
2	Dumbbell Chest Press	30 active exercise	30 recovery time	45 active exercise	15 recovery time	60 active
3	Jogging on Spot	30 active exercise	30 recovery time	45 active exercise	15 recovery time	60 active
4	Abdominal Crunch	30 active exercise	30 recovery time	45 active exercise	15 recovery time	60 active
5	Seated Dumbbell Row	30 active exercise	30 recovery time	45 active exercise	15 recovery time	60 active
6	Squat to Press	30 active exercise	30 recovery time	45 active exercise	15 recovery time	60 active
7	Dumbbell Shoulder Press	30 active exercise	30 recovery time	45 active exercise	15 recovery time	60 active
8	Opposite Arm/Leg	30 active exercise	30 recovery time	45 active exercise	15 recovery time	60 active
9	Seated Dumbbell Curl	30 active exercise	30 recovery time	45 active exercise	15 recovery time	60 active
10	Lying Hip Extension	30 active exercise	30 recovery time	45 active exercise	15 recovery time	60 active
11	Tricep Bench Dips	30 active exercise	30 recovery time	45 active exercise	15 recovery time	60 active
12	High Knees Step/Jog	30 active exercise	30 recovery time	45 active exercise	15 recovery time	60 active

Repeat twice for a total of 24 active minutes on the circuit. Recover by walking on the spot and stretching the muscle group you worked.

Resistance Training Stations   Abdominal/Lower Back Stations   Cardio Stations

We have suggested alternate exercises for most of the stations in the workout. For some stations, alternate exercises were not suggested since the exercise is a foundation exercise that should be performed routinely. However, the Truestar Workout DVD has a "special features" section that highlights a number of alternate exercises for all stations and body parts.

TIP:
Always keep your back straight when performing the squat, as rounding the back can result in serious injury. Contract your abdominals throughout the movement.

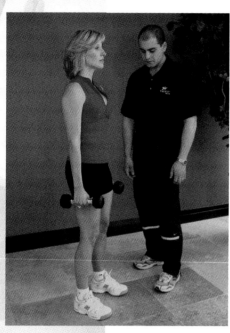

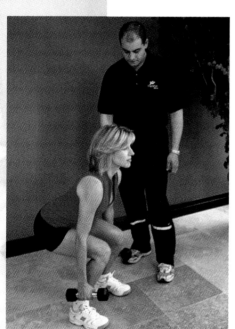

Station 1

Dumbbell Squat

STARTING POSITION
☐ Stand with your back straight and your feet shoulder width apart, with your toes pointing slightly outward.
☐ Hold the dumbbells with an overhand grip, arms extended down at your side.
☐ Contract your abdominals.

EXERCISE TECHNIQUE
☐ Lower your buttocks by bending your hips and knees until your thighs are parallel to the floor. Do not bend your knees to the point where they extend over the toes.
☐ Throughout the movement, keep your back straight and your head up. Make sure that your knees do not turn inward. Keep the weight of the dumbbells concentrated on the back of your foot, not on the toes.
☐ Pause for a moment and, without moving your back, straighten your hips and knees until you return to the starting position.
☐ Repeat the movement for the desired number of repetitions.

VARIATION
☐ You can also perform this leg-toning exercise with barbells, tubing, or medicine balls. If using a relatively light load, you can increase the intensity of this exercise by holding your thighs at a 90-degree angle for 3 to 5 seconds before returning to the starting position.

BREATHING
☐ Breathe slowly and rhythmically throughout the movement; do not hold your breath. Inhale when lowering your body, and exhale when returning to the starting position.

A shorter lead step places more emphasis on the quadriceps muscles, and a larger lead step places more emphasis on the gluteal and hamstring muscles. Hold the contraction in your thigh muscle; this will increase the tone of your thighs.

Station 1 Alternate

Static Lunge

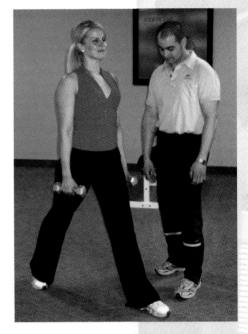

STARTING POSITION

- ☐ Stand with one foot in front of the other with your knees slightly bent.
- ☐ Grasp a dumbbell with each hand, using an overhand grip, and let your arms hang down at your sides (palms facing inward).
- ☐ Contract your abdominal muscles.

EXERCISE TECHNIQUE

- ☐ Step forward with your lead leg (stepping leg), keeping your back straight.
- ☐ Bend your lead leg (stepping leg) until your thigh is parallel to the floor and the back leg is 2 to 3 inches from the floor.
- ☐ Try not to let the knee of your lead leg travel over your toe.
- ☐ Hold that position for 3 to 5 seconds before returning to the starting position.
- ☐ Repeat the movement for the desired number of repetitions, keeping the movement fluent, slow and controlled. Perform the exercise with your other leg.

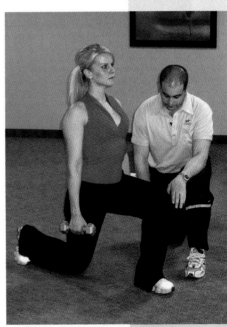

VARIATION

- ☐ Perform this exercise off of a step to generate a greater stretch and tension in the front thigh. As you get stronger, perform this exercise with resistance implements, such as medicine balls.

BREATHING

- ☐ Breathe slowly and rhythmically throughout the movement; do not hold your breath. Inhale when bending your knee and exhale when returning to the starting position.

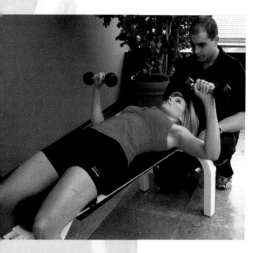

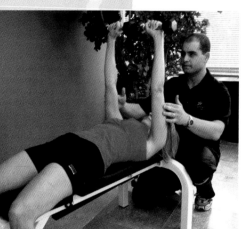

Station 2

Dumbbell Chest Press

STARTING POSITION

- ☐ Grasp two dumbbells using an overhand grip while sitting at the edge of the flat bench.
- ☐ Rest the dumbbells in an upright position on your knees.
- ☐ Lie down on the flat bench while simultaneously bringing the dumbbells to the sides of your torso at chest level.

EXERCISE TECHNIQUE

- ☐ Slowly bend your arms and lower the dumbbells until they are at either side of your chest.
- ☐ Lower the dumbbells to a point where you feel a comfortable stretch in the working muscles.
- ☐ Raise the dumbbells from the sides of the chest to the starting position.
- ☐ Do not lock your elbows during this movement. By not locking the elbows, you allow for continuous tension on the working muscles.
- ☐ Repeat the movement for the desired number of repetitions, keeping the movement fluent, slow, and controlled.

VARIATION

- ☐ Instead of raising the dumbbells straight up with palms facing forward, spice up the movement by rotating your palms inward when you are close to the top of the movement. When returning to the starting position, rotate back to a palms-forward position. This movement can also be performed with tin cans or any other easily held items.

BREATHING

- ☐ Breathe slowly and rhythmically throughout the movement; do not hold your breath. Exhale when lifting the dumbbells up and inhale when returning to the starting position.

TIP:

When raising the dumbbells, keep your chest up and focus on squeezing the chest muscles. Focus on expanding the chest muscles when returning to the starting position.

Station 2 Alternate

Incline Dumbbell Press

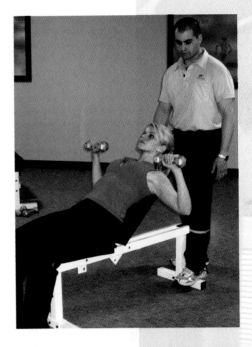

STARTING POSITION

- ☐ Grasp two dumbbells using an overhand grip while sitting on the incline bench.
- ☐ Rest the dumbbells in an upright position on your knees.
- ☐ Lie down on the incline bench while simultaneously bringing the dumbbells to the sides of your torso at chest level.

EXERCISE TECHNIQUE

- ☐ Slowly bend your arms and lower the dumbbells until they are at either side of your chest.
- ☐ Lower the dumbbells to a point where you feel a comfortable stretch in the working muscles.
- ☐ Raise the dumbbells from the sides of your chest to the starting position.
- ☐ Do not lock your elbows during this movement. By not locking the elbows, you allow for continuous tension on the working muscles.
- ☐ Repeat the movement for the desired number of repetitions, keeping the movement fluent, slow and controlled.

VARIATION

- ☐ Instead of raising the dumbbells straight up with your palms facing forward, spice up the movement by rotating your palms inward when you are close to the top of the movement. When returning to the starting position, rotate back to a palms-forward position. This movement can also be performed with tin cans or any other easily held items.

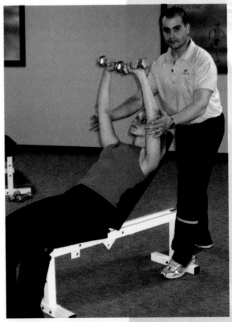

BREATHING

- ☐ Breathe slowly and rhythmically throughout the movement; do not hold your breath. Exhale when lifting the dumbbells up and inhale when returning to the starting position.

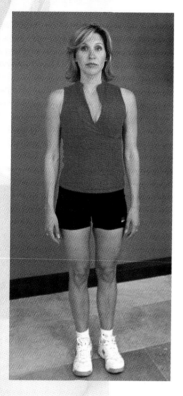
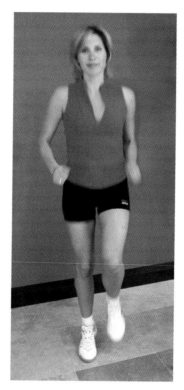

Cardio: Jogging on Spot

STARTING POSITION

- From a standing position, begin to jog on the spot. Try to coordinate your arms and legs so your opposite arm and leg are forward at the same time.

EXERCISE TECHNIQUE

- Maintain good posture by keeping your head and chest up. Lifting your knees high, toward your chest, will increase the difficulty of this movement.

VARIATION

- Perform exercise with high knees and faster to minimize foot contact on the ground.

BREATHING

- Breathe slowly and rhythmically throughout the entire movement.

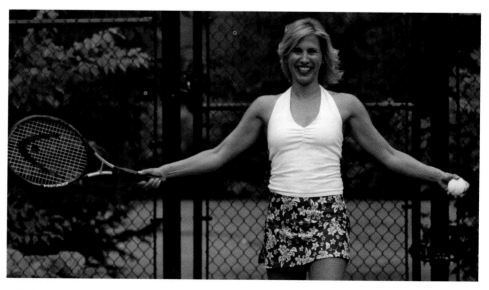

When bending forward, try to squeeze your belly button between your upper and lower abdominals. Try not to initiate the movement from your hips, as this will place more emphasis on the hip flexor muscles than on the abdominals.

Station 4

Abdominal Crunch

STARTING POSITION
- ☐ Lie flat on the mat with your knees bent and your feet on the floor.
- ☐ Place your hands at shoulder level.

EXERCISE TECHNIQUE
- ☐ Curl your upper abdominals to raise your head and shoulders from the mat.
- ☐ When your upper abdominal muscles are fully contracted, pause briefly and return to the starting position.
- ☐ To keep tension on your working muscles; do not allow your upper back and shoulders to make contact with the mat.
- ☐ Repeat the movement for the desired number of repetitions.

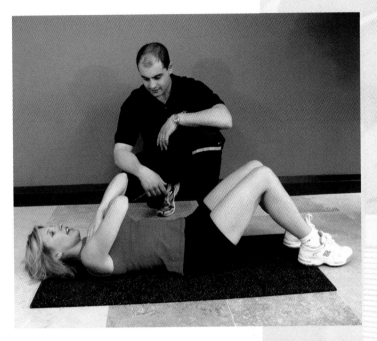

VARIATION
- ☐ Change your hand placement to change the difficulty of the exercise. Placing the arms across the body is for beginners, placing the hands and arms behind the head is for intermediates, and extending the arms and hands over the head is for advanced.
  If you do not wish to increase the number of repetitions or sets, the difficulty of the exercise can be increased by placing a load — such as a medicine ball or a light weight — on your chest area.

BREATHING
- ☐ Breathe slowly and rhythmically throughout the movement; do not hold your breath. Exhale when squeezing your abdominals and inhale when returning to the starting position.

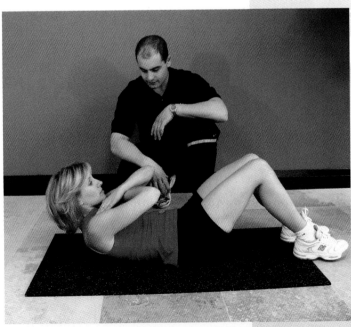

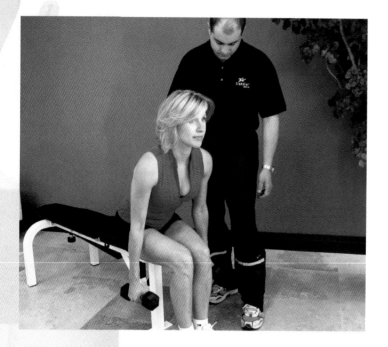

Seated Dumbbell Row

STARTING POSITION

☐ Sit at the edge of a bench or chair with feet shoulder width part and dumbbells at the side of the body palms facing in.

☐ Slightly bend you upper body forward to approximately a 45-degree angle and contract the abdominal muscles.

EXERCISE TECHNIQUE

☐ Keeping your upper body bent, pull the dumbbells upward and keep your elbows as close to the body as possible. Stop the upward movement when the elbow is at approximately a 90-degree angle. Imagine a pencil between your shoulder blades and squeeze the pencil as you pull the dumbbells upward.

☐ Slowly return the dumbbells to the starting position and repeat the movement.

VARIATION

☐ Perform the movement one arm at a time for variety or alternate right and left arm for the duration of the station time. You can also change the hand position to a palm-forward facing direction.

BREATHING

☐ Breathe slowly and rhythmically throughout the movement.

☐ Breathe out when raising the dumbbells and breathe in when returning to starting position.

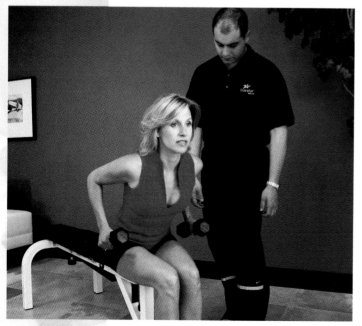

TIP:

It is important that you do not move the hips while performing the exercise. Do not over extend the dumbbell and choose a weight that feels comfortable and secure. Also, if you are utilizing dumbbells that snap together, make sure that the weights on the dumbbell are tightly held in place before performing this exercise.

Station 5 Alternate

Dumbbell Pullover

STARTING POSITION

- ☐ Grasp a dumbbell by placing the palms against the inner portion of one end of the dumbbell.
- ☐ Lie on a flat bench and lift the dumbbell over your forehead. Hold it at arms length.
- ☐ Your knees are bent slightly less than 90 degrees.

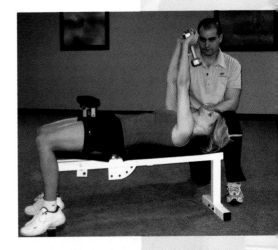

EXERCISE TECHNIQUE

- ☐ Lower the dumbbell in an arc fashion until you feel a comfortable stretch in your upper back and shoulders or until your elbows are in line with your shoulders. Make sure your hips are not raised or lowered throughout the movement.
- ☐ Hold the extended stretch for 1 to 2 seconds, before you pull the dumbbell back up in the same arc-like fashion over into the starting position, approximately above the upper chest area. Maintain a slight bend in the elbow. Contract the chest, upper back, and abdominal muscles when performing the movement.
- ☐ Complete the exercise until the desired number of repetitions is reached.

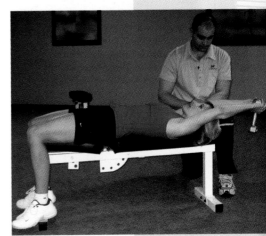

VARIATION

- ☐ This exercise can also be performed by lying across a bench. This exercise can be performed with a barbell, weighted bar, or medicine ball, as well.

BREATHING

- ☐ Breathe slowly and rhythmically throughout the movement; do not hold your breath. Breathe in when lowering the dumbbell and breathe out when returning the dumbbell to the starting position.

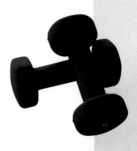

Do not let your knees fall inward and never let them pass over your toes. Keep your head up at all times and do not round your back. Contracting your abdominal muscles will help you maintain a proper posture. Perform this exercise rhythmically.

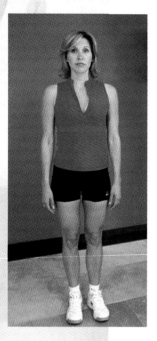
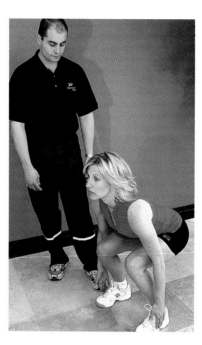

Station 6

Cardio: Squat to Press

STARTING POSITION

☐ Stand up straight with your feet shoulder width apart, and your toes pointed forward. Imagine holding a dumbbell in each hand at the side of your body.

EXERCISE TECHNIQUE

☐ Bend at the hips and knees, bringing your buttocks toward the floor. Keep your back straight throughout the movement and make sure that your knees do not pass over your toes. Lower your body to a 90-degree angle (your thighs should be parallel to the floor) and pause for a moment. Without moving your back, straighten your hips and knees to the starting position. Keep your weight on the back of your feet, not on your toes.

☐ Extend your arms and raise your hands so that they meet above your head. Lower your hands and begin the next repetition.

VARIATION

☐ Perform this exercise with body weight alone or with dumbbells or medicine balls.

BREATHING

☐ Breathe out as you extend your arms overhead and breathe in when returning to the bending position.

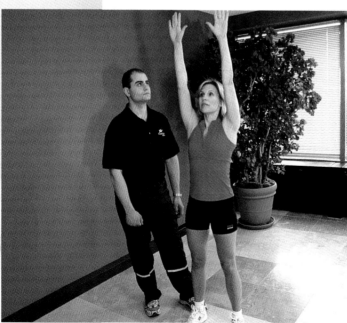

TIP:

Avoid arching or overextending your back. Do not lock your elbows.

Contract your abdominal muscles throughout the movement.

Station 7

Dumbbell Shoulder Press

STARTING POSITION

☐ Sit with your feet shoulder width apart. Grasp two dumbbells with an overhand grip, palms facing forward, and lift them to your shoulders.

EXERCISE TECHNIQUE

☐ Keep your head in line with your body and your eyes focused straight ahead. Extend your arms and press the dumbbells upward.

☐ The dumbbells should meet at the end of the movement, above your head, and your palms should remain facing forward.

☐ Return to the starting position.

VARIATION

☐ Your palms may face each other in the beginning and final position. You may also try alternating arms.

BREATHING

☐ Exhale as you press the dumbbells upward and inhale as you return to the starting position. Do not hold your breath at any time.

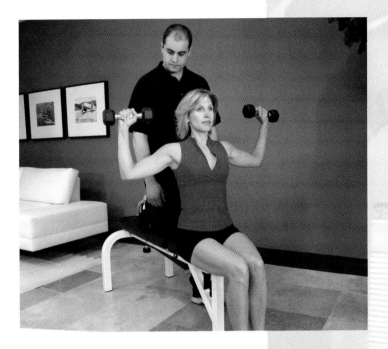

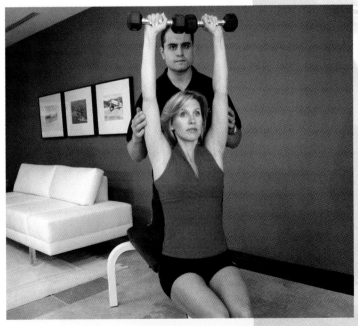

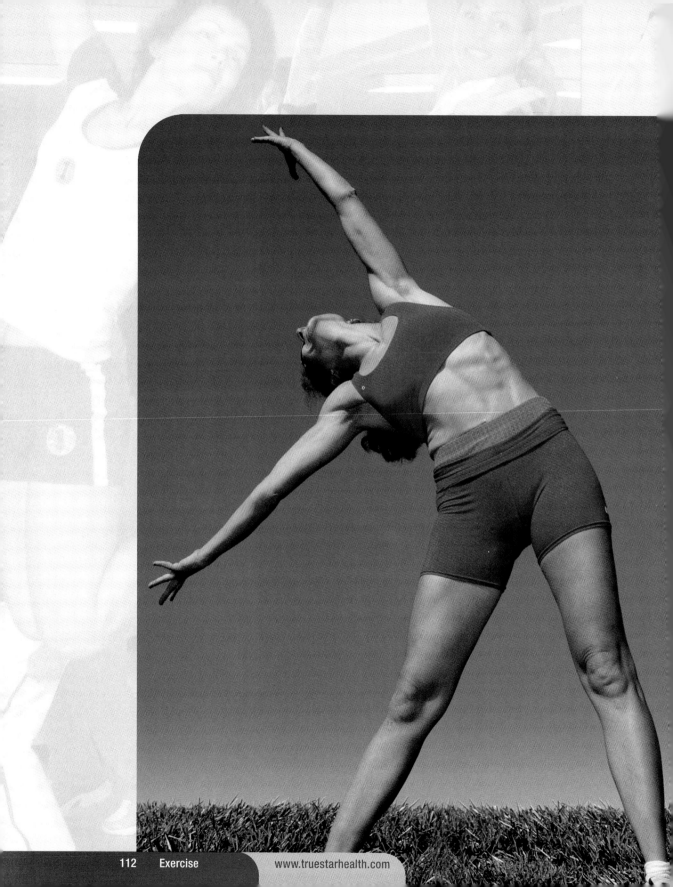

TIP:
Contract your abdomen, lower back, and buttocks muscles throughout
the entire movement.

Station 8

Opposite Arm/Leg

STARTING POSITION

☐ Lie down flat on your stomach with your
arms extended directly in front of you and
palms down. You legs are extended straight
behind you.

☐ Place your chin comfortably on the floor.

EXERCISE TECHNIQUE

☐ Extend your right arm and left leg simultaneously a few inches off the floor. When
your reach the top of the movement, hold
the position for 1 to 2 seconds before
slowly returning to the starting position.
Do not extend the arm above shoulder
height or the leg above hip height.

☐ Repeat the movement with the left arm
and right leg.

☐ Alternate the movement between both
sets of legs and arms until the desired
number of repetitions is completed.

VARIATION

☐ You can alternate this exercise by
performing it on your knees. If you
experience problems lifting your arm
and leg combination at the same time,
start off by first lifting the arm into
position and follow with the leg.

BREATHING

☐ Breathe slowly and rhythmically throughout the movement; do not hold your
breath. Breathe out when extending
the arm and leg upward and breathe in
when returning the limbs to the starting
position.

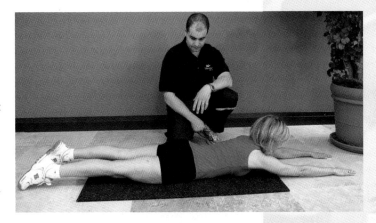

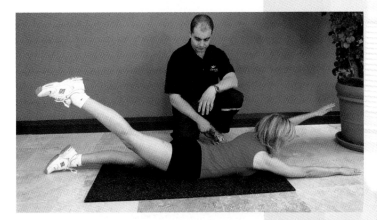

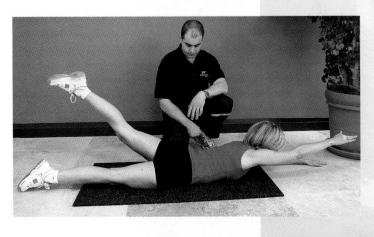

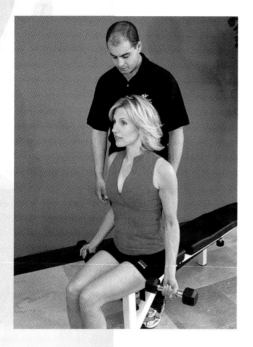

Seated Dumbbell Curl

STARTING POSITION

☐ Grasp the dumbbells using an underhand grip (palms forward).

☐ Sit on a bench with your back straight, knees bent, and feet shoulder width apart.

☐ Arms are fully extended and the dumbbells are hanging straight down at your sides.

EXERCISE TECHNIQUE

☐ Initiate the movement by bending at the elbow, curling the right dumbbell up, toward your shoulder.

☐ Slowly lower the dumbbell to the starting position and repeat the movement with the left arm.

☐ Continue alternating arms until the desired number of repetitions is complete.

VARIATION

☐ This exercise can also be performed with both arms moving at the same time. You may begin your set by performing a bilateral dumbbell curl and finish the set by alternating.

☐ Your palm can remain in a forward-facing position throughout the entire movement or be positioned in, toward the thigh, as the dumbbell is lowered. When curling the dumbbell for the next repetition, the palm will be facing forward on the up motion.

BREATHING

☐ Exhale when curling the dumbbell up and inhale when relaxing the dumbbell down. Breathe in a slow and rhythmic manner throughout the movement; do not hold your breath.

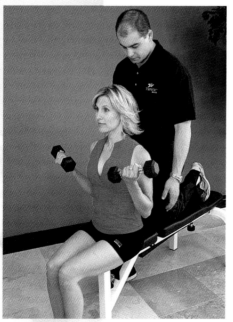

Squeeze your biceps at the top of the movement and keep your elbows tucked in to your torso. Constant outward movement of the elbows may be an indication the weight is too heavy.

Station 9 Alternate

Incline Dumbbell Curl

STARTING POSITION
- ☐ Lie down on the incline bench with your back pressed firmly against the padding.
- ☐ Hold a dumbbell in each hand using an underhand grip (palms facing up), and rest your arms down by your sides.

EXERCISE TECHNIQUE
- ☐ Flex at the elbow and curl the dumbbells up, toward your shoulders.
- ☐ Hold this position for a moment, then slowly lower the dumbbells to the starting position. You may perform this exercise one arm at a time or both arms together.
- ☐ Repeat the movement for the desired number of repetitions.

VARIATION
- ☐ Change the angle of the bench.

BREATHING
- ☐ Breathe slowly and rhythmically throughout the movement; do not hold your breath. Exhale as you curl the weight upward and inhale as you return to the starting position.

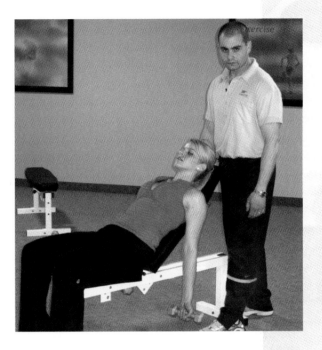

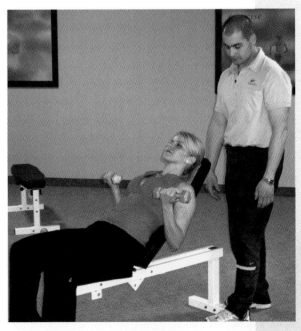

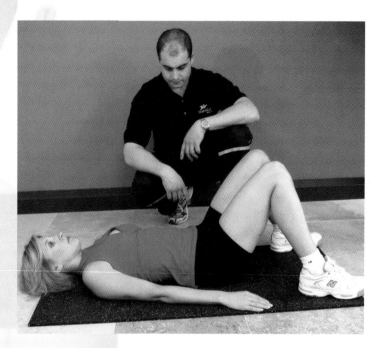

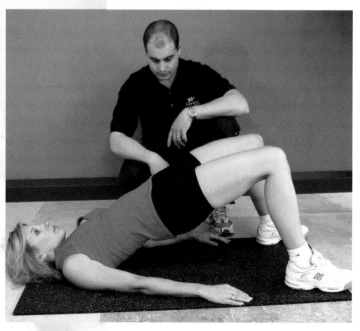

Station 10

Lying Hip Extension

STARTING POSITION

☐ Lie on your back on the floor with your knees bent and your arms positioned at your side (palms facing down).

EXERCISE TECHNIQUE

☐ Raise your hips off the floor until you feel maximum contraction in your buttocks muscles.

☐ Hold the contraction for 1 to 2 seconds before returning to the starting position.

☐ Repeat the movement for the desired number of repetitions, keeping the movement fluent, slow, and controlled.

VARIATION

☐ Point your toes in different directions to stimulate different areas of the glutes. Pointing your toes outward will place more emphasis on the inner buttocks, and pointing your toes inward will place more emphasis on the outer buttocks region. For an advanced variation, raise your heels off the floor when you are raising your hips upward. This variation will simultaneously stimulate your calf muscles.

☐ Place dumbbell on your hips to increase the resistance.

BREATHING

☐ Breathe slowly and rhythmically throughout the movement; do not hold your breath.

☐ Exhale when extending upward and inhale when returning to the starting position.

Station 10 Alternate

Arm Reach

STARTING POSITION

☐ Sit with your knees bent at a 90-degree angle and your back straight. Lean slightly back until you feel the contraction in your abdominal muscles. Your upper body should be at approximately a 45-degree angle.

☐ Extend both arms in front of your body.

EXERCISE TECHNIQUE

☐ Imagine a wall with a shelf on each side of your body and slowly reach your right arm towards the left shelf by slightly rotating at your waist. You should feel tension on the side of your abdominal muscles.

☐ Return to the starting position and repeat with the left arm. Make sure to keep your abdominals tight and upper body back for the duration of the exercise.

VARIATION

☐ Keeping your upper body in a leaning position, thus contracting your abdominal muscles, and clasp your hands together in front of your body and keep a slight bend in the elbows. Imagine a rainbow in front of your body and rotate your hand from one end of the rainbow to the other end. Imagine the height of the rainbow at your forehead level.

BREATHING

☐ Breathe slowly and rhythmically throughout the movement; do not hold your breath.

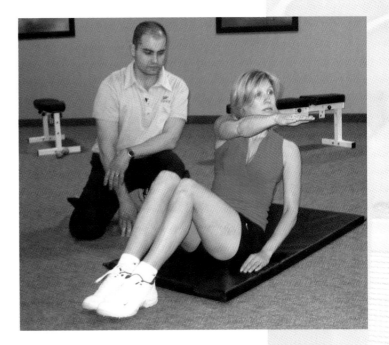

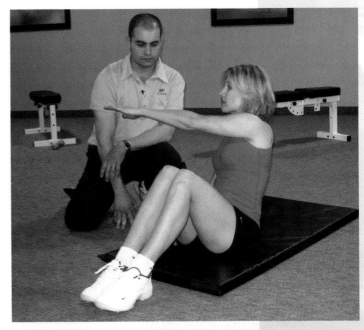

TIP:
Bend your elbows at a 90-degree angle; stretching the shoulder muscles
further may result in injury.

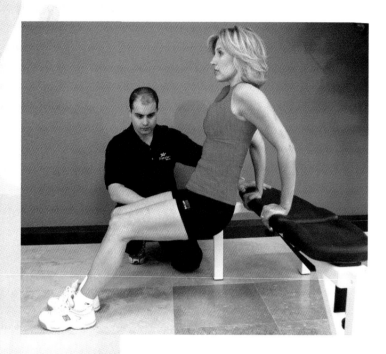

Station 11

Tricep Bench Dips

STARTING POSITION

☐ Place your hands shoulder width apart
on the edge of the bench, and place your
heels on the floor, with your knees bent.

☐ Extend your arms completely and hold
this position.

☐ Do not lock out the elbows.

EXERCISE TECHNIQUE

☐ Initiate the movement by slowly bending
your arms until your elbow is at a
90-degree angle.

☐ Slowly push back up to the starting position by straightening your arms. Repeat
the movement for the desired number of
repetitions.

VARIATION

☐ Add resistance to the exercise by placing
a dumbbell or a weight plate on the front
of your thighs when performing the
movement.

☐ Extend your legs to increase the intensity
of the movement. You can also raise one
leg off the floor or place both legs on a
bench to increase the intensity further.

BREATHING

☐ Exhale as you extend upward and inhale
as you return to the starting position.
Breathe slowly and rhythmically
throughout the movement; do not hold
your breath.

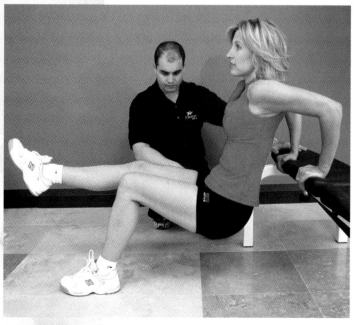

Cardio: High Knees Step/Jog

STARTING POSITION

☐ From a standing position, begin to jog on the spot. Try to coordinate your arms and legs so your opposite arm and leg are forward at the same time.

EXERCISE TECHNIQUE

☐ As a guide, place your hands palms down at hip level and attempt to touch your knees to your hands with every upward movement. The goal is to pull the knee up towards the hip.

VARIATION

☐ Slow down the speed of the movement and attempt to increase the range of motion by which you raise the leg off the ground.

BREATHING

☐ Breathe slowly and rhythmically throughout the movement.

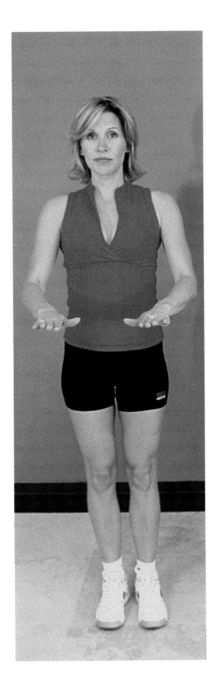
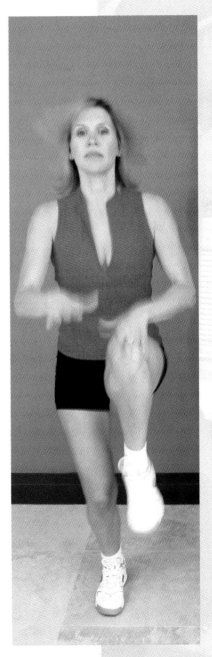

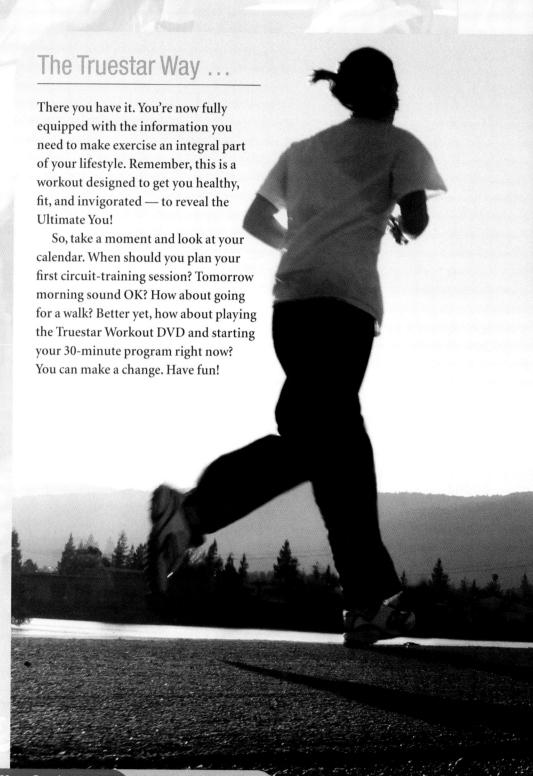

The Truestar Way …

There you have it. You're now fully equipped with the information you need to make exercise an integral part of your lifestyle. Remember, this is a workout designed to get you healthy, fit, and invigorated — to reveal the Ultimate You!

So, take a moment and look at your calendar. When should you plan your first circuit-training session? Tomorrow morning sound OK? How about going for a walk? Better yet, how about playing the Truestar Workout DVD and starting your 30-minute program right now? You can make a change. Have fun!

"The longest journey starts with a single step."
Lao Tse

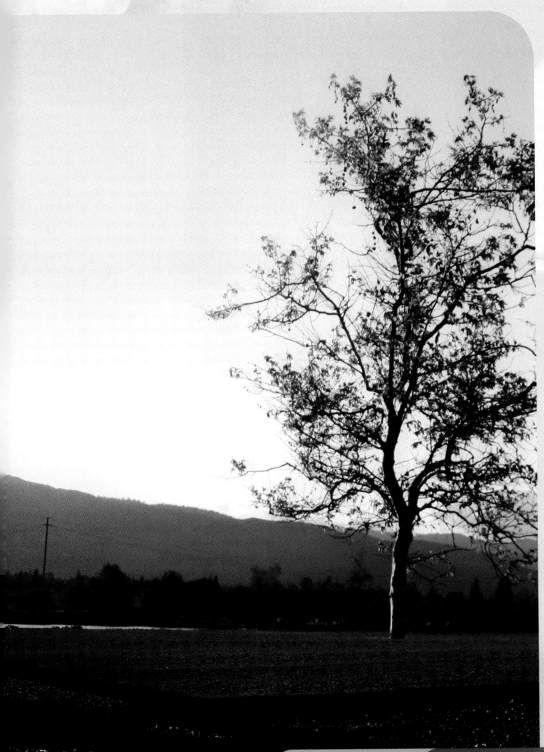

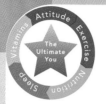

I feel like a different person inside …

How Truestar Way Changed My Life

Truestar for Women, I would really like to thank you for changing my life forever! Thank you for caring enough to get together a team of professionals who know what to do and how to do it!

Your total program of nutrition, exercise, vitamins, attitude, and sleep has been a life-changing experience for me — and I love it! I am so grateful that your program helped me change my life in terms of my physical activity level and the way I look at food. The coaches and staff at my local Truestar Women's Nutrition and Fitness Center are so supportive and helpful and make me feel like I always want to be at Truestar. I love them all.

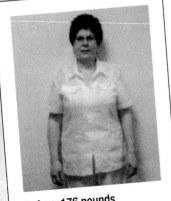

Before: 176 pounds

I feel alive and in control of who I am.

I have lost 47 pounds and 46.5 inches and have gone down 4 sizes since joining Truestar. I feel so great about myself and about the way I look.

But even more important to me than my physical appearance is the way I feel inside. I am so focused about taking my supplements, doing my exercises 5 to 6 days a week, and eating properly now that I feel like a different person inside. I feel alive and in control of who I am. I needed the Truestar program to change my life. It fits into my life and will always help me make healthier choices. I have tried many programs out there, but the Truestar program is the only one out with a total package that works.

When people ask me how I lost all my weight, I tell them that I joined a great team. I love the way I look and feel and love going to the Truestar Center. It's also great that all the other members are women only!

I will continue working hard to strive for positive changes in my life. Thank you from the bottom of my heart.

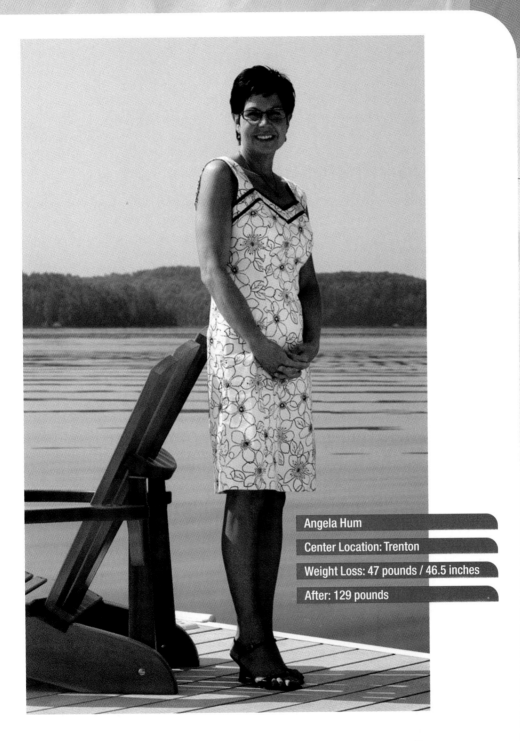

When people ask me how I lost all my weight, I tell them that I joined a great team!

Angela Hum

Center Location: Trenton

Weight Loss: 47 pounds / 46.5 inches

After: 129 pounds

Vitamins

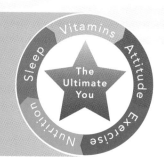

Bring on the Vitamins!

Tim Mulcahy

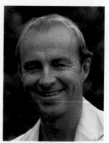

Tim Mulcahy

After nutrition and exercise, vitamins were my next discovery for maintaining a high energy level and optimal health, something I needed in my career as a direct marketing entrepreneur and in my home life as a full-time father and husband. The discovery that I needed something more than good food and regular exercise to prevent an afternoon energy lag, common to many people as they begin to age, came when I was 28. I tried taking a high-potency multivitamin that contained high levels of vitamin B, with the result that my afternoon lag was almost unnoticeable, if not completely gone.

This whetted my appetite to learn more about vitamins and supplements. I soon became a health-food store junkie and started to take MSM for my knees, which bothered me after exercising. I took extra vitamin C, some green products, and co-enzyme Q 10, also adding protein powder to my drinks. This vitamin plan seemed to work, as I learned one day when I forgot to take my vitamins. I was sitting in my office at around 4:00 p.m. and wondered why I was still feeling tired. I reviewed my day — I exercised in the morning, I slept well, and I ate fairly well (at least I thought so). Then it dawned on me — I forgot my vitamins at home that morning.

That's a concern I don't have these days — at the Truestar Health office we happen to be fairly well stocked with a full line of specially formulated Truestar vitamins to keep your energy levels high and assist with weight loss. Without the vitamin regimen that I'm currently following, I'm sure I would get ill much more frequently (currently that is rare, thank God) and I would be a target for more serious illness. I tend to burn the candle at both ends. Building new businesses, which I've done at least a dozen times in the last 20 years, takes its toll in the stress department.

Here's what I now take daily from the Truestar Health Professional Series of supplements:

> "Supplementing an intelligent diet is an intelligent thing."
> Dr. Margo Feldweis

- TrueBasics for Men: High-potency multivitamin + calcium-magnesium + omega-3 fish oil + 8 tocopherol vitamin E + grape seed extract), daily
- TrueLean, 2 tablets, twice daily
- TrueCraving Control, 4-8 tablets daily
- TrueCell: Alpha lipoic acid and CoQ10, twice daily
- TrueMSM, 1000 mg, daily
- TrueC, 6000 mg, daily
- TrueProtect: A,C, E, selenium, zinc, twice daily
- TrueB: High-potency B complex, twice daily
- TrueBoost: L-tyrosine, 2000 mg, daily
- TrueFlow: L-arginine, 1000 mg daily
- TrueAllerfree, daily
- TrueOmega: High-grade fish oil, 2000 mg, daily
- TrueZZZs: melatonin, three times weekly
- TrueStrength: Protein powder
- Acidophilus Lactobacillus

Vitamins and supplements are my form of life insurance. While I am alive in this amazing world, I want to feel my very best and have the highest possible energy level while boosting my immune system to protect my body from disease.

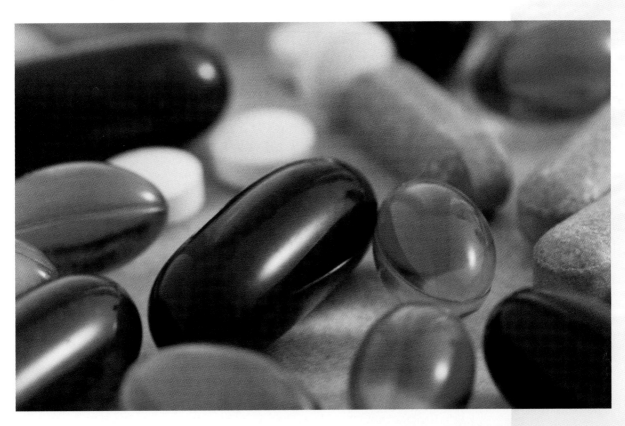

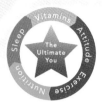

Vitamins … the Truestar Way

Dr Natasha Turner, ND
Vice-President, Natural Medicine

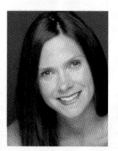

Natasha Turner

Most people take vitamins to boost energy and prevent illness, while others believe it will help them live longer and healthier lives.

Take heed — as you begin this leg in your journey toward optimal health, trust me, you will get hooked. I remember the time when I took only one multivitamin in the morning. Now, I take so many vitamin pills, a close friend of mine thinks I rattle when I walk!

Like the other principles of the Truestar way — nutrition, exercise, attitude, and sleep — vitamins lead to optimal health and lifelong wellness. They are especially effective in preventing illness and preserving good health.

The Vitamin Boom

More people are taking nutritional supplements than ever before. It is estimated that over 100 million Americans take vitamins on a regular basis. Almost half of the Canadian population takes supplements daily, with 68% of people over 65 doing so regularly.

Not only are more people taking vitamins, but many people are also adding more vitamins to their daily regimen. The nutritional supplement market is expected to grow by 20% per year in Canada and by 30% in the United States. This may leave you wondering why people are taking vitamins and why they are taking more vitamins than before. Is it just the newest health craze? We know it's not.

Most people take vitamins to boost energy and prevent illness, while others believe it will help them live longer and healthier lives. Others enjoy the empowering feeling associated with doing something every day to take better care of themselves through the practice of preventive medicine.

Your Health Bank

Simply put, we believe the best way to think of vitamins and supplements is as a deposit in a savings account at your 'health' bank for use later in life or as the

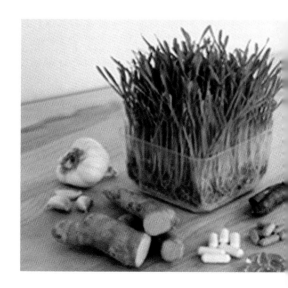

Log on to www.truestarhealth.com to create a personal vitamin plan based on your weight-loss goals, physical activity level, and current health status.

premium for a 'health' insurance plan. Your deposit will pay compound interest on the investment and the insurance plan we hope will never be needed!

Here, we'll provide you with the basics you need to know about vitamins — how to take them, when, where, why, and so on. Heads up, though, because we pres-ent a lot of information in a short amount of space. While we don't expect you will be able to recall this information freely, we suggest you keep it handy for quick reference as your wellness guide. Welcome to the fabulous world of Truestar nutritional supplements!

What Are Vitamins?

Vitamins are micronutrients we ingest from food. They are essential to health. They promote normal growth, help to heal injuries, fight off infections, regulate proper metabolism, remove waste, and protect against certain diseases, such as cancer and heart disease. They are the building blocks for the majority of chemical reactions in our bodies. Vitamins combine with amino acids and minerals to produce enzymes (which speed up internal chemical reactions) and hormones (chemical messengers which regulate organ functions and activities, including heart rate, blood pressure, and glucose levels). A deficiency of just one vitamin can cause widespread harm in the body.

While we often group all micro-nutrients and nutritional supplements under the heading of 'vitamins', they are chemically distinct from minerals, amino acids, essential fatty acids, and enzymes, for example. Still, vitamins often work synergistically with these other micronutrients.

TWO GROUPS OF VITAMINS

☐ Fat Soluble

Fat-soluble vitamins, such as vita-min A, D, E, and K, can be stored in the body, mostly in fatty tissue and in the liver. Because they can be stored, you do not always need a steady supply of these vitamins, but they can build to toxic levels if you consume too much.

☐ Water Soluble

Water-soluble vitamins, such as vitamin C and the B vitamins, do not stay in the body long. Since they dissolve in water, any traces of the vitamins that the body does not need will be carried away in waste. Because they cannot be stored, we need to receive a healthy supply of these vitamins every day. Except in cases of massive over-dosing, water-soluble vitamins rarely reach toxic levels.

Simply put, we believe the best way to think of vitamins and supplements is as a deposit in a savings account at your 'health' bank for use later in life or as the premium for a 'health' insurance plan.

What Are Minerals?

Like vitamins, minerals are micronutrients essential to our health. Every living cell requires minerals for proper structure and function. Minerals are needed for healthy bone, muscle tone, and nerves, for proper composition of body fluids, for strong function of the cardiovascular system, and for the formation of blood. Like vitamins, they are important coenzymes or catalysts, involved in the production of energy, normal growth, and healing.

Each of the minerals is interdependent upon the other, so a balance must be maintained for proper chemical functioning of the body.

TWO GROUPS OF MINERALS

□ Macro Minerals

Macro or bulk minerals, such as potassium, magnesium, calcium, sodium, and phosphorous, are needed by the body in higher amounts than micro minerals.

□ Micro Minerals

Also called trace minerals, micro minerals include boron, zinc, chromium, copper, germanium, silicon, sulfur, vanadium, iodine, manganese, molybdenum, iron, and selenium. They are required in a much lower dosage than macro minerals, but their role in maintaining good health is equally essential.

Mineral Balance

Each of the minerals is interdependent upon the other, so a balance must be maintained for proper chemical functioning of the body. If the initial deficiency or excess of one mineral is not corrected, an illness may result.

Like the fat-soluble vitamins, minerals are absorbed and stored in the body's tissues; therefore, it is possible to develop mineral toxicity if large quantities are consumed over long periods of time. This is rare, however. The most common excess condition tends to occur with iron.

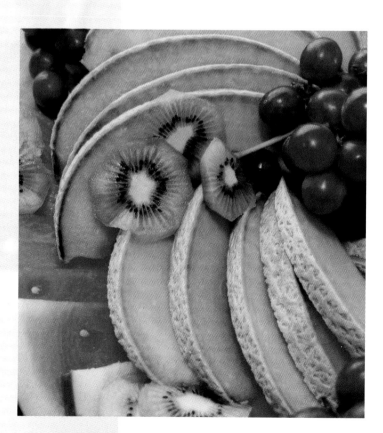

Some minerals, once in the blood stream, compete with others for absorption and transport into cells. Due to this process, mineral supplements should always be taken in balanced amounts, unless a depletion of one particular mineral is desired. For example, too much zinc can cause a reduction in copper levels, and excess magnesium can deplete calcium.

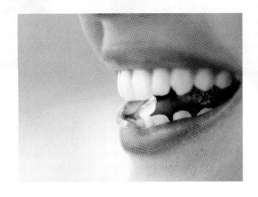

Many people have copper toxicity effectively treated by ingesting high levels of zinc to cause increased copper loss.

Vitamin and Mineral Deficiencies

We often ask ourselves, "Do I really need to take supplements if I eat well?" The answer is "yes" if you desire optimal health. Supplements are necessary to achieve optimal health for two reasons: first, because a deficiency of just one nutrient leaves you at risk of illness, and second, because nutrient supplements can help to prevent illness. If you think you eat well and don't require supplements, keep reading — you may be surprised to realize the opposite is true.

Nutrient-Depleted Soils

During the past 50 years or so, our food supply has become increasingly nutrient-deficient and unbalanced because of intensive farming practices. We have exhausted our soil and upset natural nutrient balances. These problems are, of course, reflected in the foods we eat grown in this soil. To compound the problem, nutrients are lost in food processing — preserving, drying, freezing, and packaging. For example, processing whole grains into white flour to increase their shelf-life strips out required vitamins and minerals, such as vitamin B-1 (thiamine) and vitamin B-3 (niacin), leaving us at risk for deficiency diseases, such as pellagra (vitamin B-3) and beri-beri (vitamin B-1). To compensate for these deficiencies, food manufacturers 'fortify' these foods with the vitamins and minerals stripped out during processing.

We have exhausted our soil and upset natural nutrient balances.

Poor Dietary Habits

Since the body cannot produce vitamins on its own, we must get them from the foods we eat. Unfortunately, we rarely eat a wide enough variety of food to get healthy levels of all necessary vitamins. Although it's best to get as many vitamins as possible from natural foods, supplements are often required to keep the body functioning properly.

Environmental and Lifestyle Stress

The *Journal of the American Medical Association* reported that elderly people, vegans, alcohol-dependent individuals, and patients with malabsorption conditions are at higher risk of inadequate intake or absorption of several vitamins. Pollution, stress, sleep deprivation, exercise, family history, health risk factors, illness, and even coffee consumption can all cause an increased need for vitamin supplementation.

Aging

Elderly and hospitalized patients are particularly at risk for nutrient deficiencies. In a 30-month study of 800 American patients who were admitted to hospital for conditions not normally associated with malnutrition (pneumonia and hip fracture, for example), blood tests found 55% to be malnourished. The malnourished surgical patients stayed in the hospital an average of 5 days longer than the adequately nourished patients. In a study of 402 elderly Europeans living at home, the nutrient content of their diet was found to be low: folic acid intake was low in 100% of those studied, zinc in 87%, vitamin B-6 in 83%, and vitamin D in 62%.

Medications

Many prescription and over-the-counter medications deplete our store of vitamins and minerals. While these drugs may be beneficial in the treatment of a disease condition, they may come with a nutritional cost. For example, the birth control pill causes a decrease in zinc, folic acid, vitamin B-12, vitamin B-6, and vitamin C.

Elderly and hospitalized patients are particularly at risk for nutrient deficiencies.

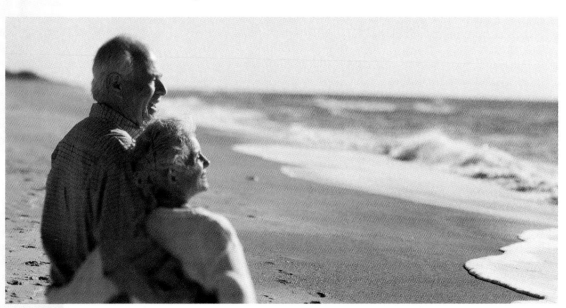

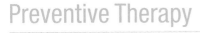

Aspirin causes increased loss of vitamin C. H_2 blocker drugs, which are used to treat gastric ulcers, deplete vitamin B-12, vitamin D, folic acid, iron, zinc, and calcium.

The www.truestarhealth.com online vitamin section provides a comprehensive discussion of possible harmful interactions between supplements and drugs, with information about nutrient depletions caused by any medications you are taking. Our system identifies products you should not be taking (contraindicated) and how to supplement properly for drug-induced nutrient depletions.

Longer Life Span

In general, we live longer than we did a century ago. We now require nutrients over a longer period of time so that we may age in good health. As we age, our body slows down. Cellular function, organ function, metabolism, and repair processes are not as optimal as they were in our early twenties. Our digestive function decreases and so does our ability to take in vitamins in minerals. Vitamins and supplements provide extra fuel for the long journey ahead.

A complete multivitamin is the only effective way to ensure that all essential bodily processes take place. Don't leave yourself lacking and more susceptible to infections and diseases.

> A complete multivitamin is the only effective way to ensure that all essential bodily processes take place. Don't leave yourself lacking and more susceptible to infections and diseases.

Preventive Therapy

Vitamin and mineral supplements not only satisfy nutrient deficiencies and rectify nutrient imbalances, they also serve as preventive therapy. Supplementing your diet with certain vitamins and minerals may significantly reduce your risk of future health concerns. For example, taking folic acid can prevent neural tube defect in the fetus. Vitamin B-6 and vitamin B-12 optimize homocysteine metabolism and lower coronary heart disease risk. Vitamin E, selenium, and lycopene may decrease the risk of prostate cancer, while vitamin D, when taken with calcium, is associated with decreased occurrence of osteoporosis. Simply taking vitamin E and vitamin C each day can reduce your risk of Alzheimer's disease by 58%. Considering that by the time we are 80 years old, 50% of us may develop Alzheimer's, this should be good news to all of us.

By educating yourself in the use of vitamins and supplements, you can support the treatment of certain medical conditions safely without side effects. For example, mild cervical dysplasia or abnormal PAP test results can be treated effectively with folic acid supplements. Certain vitamins may be prescribed by your licensed healthcare provider to reduce symptoms or to treat disease, such as iron to treat anemia or calcium and vitamin D to treat loss of bone density.

Log on to www.truestarhealth.com to create a personal vitamin plan based on your weight-loss goals, physical activity level, and current health status.

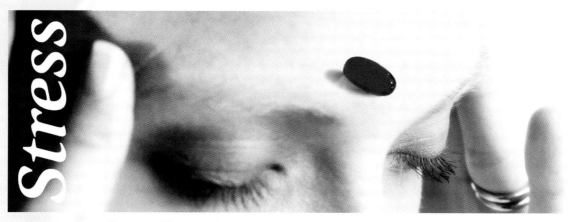

Stress

The basic supplements you need to take daily are calcium-magnesium, fish oils, mixed vitamin E, and antioxidants, such as vitamin C or grapeseed extract, along with a multivitamin.

Prevent Weight Gain

Our bodies need the proper balance of vitamins and minerals each day to support a healthy metabolism. For example, a deficiency of B vitamins may reduce the ability to process carbohydrates properly, causing weight gain. Our thyroid gland, which governs metabolism, needs nutrients, such as selenium, iodine, zinc, tyrosine, and vitamin D, to make the thyroid hormone that maintains metabolic rate. Without these nutrients, we tend to gain weight and experience fatigue.

The basic supplements you need to take daily are calcium-magnesium, fish oils, mixed vitamin E, and antioxidants, such as vitamin C or grapeseed extract, along with a multivitamin.

Increase Energy Levels

One of the first improvements many people notice when they begin taking vitamins is higher energy levels throughout the day. The 3:00 to 4:00 p.m. energy 'lag' or 'slump' can be prevented with the proper intake of vitamins, especially B vitamins. A deficiency may cause our normal cellular processes to slow down, eventually resulting in the physical symptom of fatigue. Magnesium, for example, is necessary for over 300 enzymatic reactions in the body. Imagine if you do not have enough magnesium. Your body will slow down on a cellular level, eventually resulting in the physical manifestation of fatigue. A decrease in energy is often the first sign that something is out of balance. Most people ignore this sign for years.

Eliminate Cravings

Cravings are sometimes an indication that your body needs nutrients. For instance, low levels of magnesium are associated with chocolate cravings, and a deficiency of chromium or the amino acid glutamine can increase cravings for sugar. To ward off these cravings and the health conditions associated with them, take your supplements.

Decrease Stress

Some studies indicate that our vitamin C stores in the adrenal glands deplete within 20 to 30 minutes of being under stress. Our adrenal glands are also called the 'stress' glands because they release the short-term stress hormone adrenalin and the long-term stress hormone cortisol in response to physical, mental, and emotional stress. Take your vitamin C if you are under stress at work or at home to avoid the risk of having suboptimal levels. Because vitamin C is also a potent antioxidant, immune-supporting nutrient, and component of healthy collagen synthesis for skin and other body tissues, you want to make sure you get enough each day.

Improve Memory

Poor concentration — poor attention span? If you need to be more focused, take your fish oils daily. Supplements of fish oils, especially those higher in DHA, protect the brain from elevated levels of stress hormones linked to memory loss. Magnesium and zinc help with learning and attention, making them essential supplements for good concentration and awareness. Low iron levels have also been associated with poor concentration and learning in children. And don't forget the benefit of daily use of vitamin C and vitamin E supplements for reducing the risk of Alzheimer's.

Elevate Mood

If you are not meeting your nutritional needs, your body cannot make hormones, such as serotonin, which affects your mood, memory, cravings, appetite, and sleep. Taking supplements may assist in the prevention of depression, insomnia, and carbohydrate cravings by providing sufficient vitamin B-6 and the amino acid tryptophan required for the creation of serotonin. Tyrosine and phenylalanine are important for the production of dopamine, which is also involved in appetite regulation, addictions, metabolic rate, and mood.

Many people who take supplements also report feelings of empowerment as they are doing something proactively each day to maintain their health and promote wellness.

Take your vitamin C if you are under stress at work or at home to avoid the risk of having suboptimal levels.

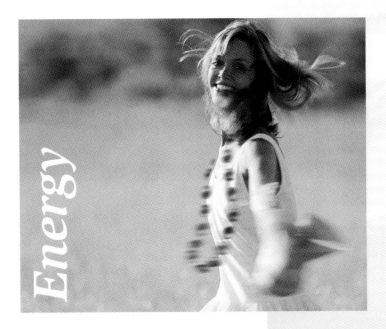

Energy

Boost Libido

A healthy libido is a sign of good health. Your sex drive is a basic human need like hunger — without it, something is wrong. Remember, the basic laws of nature entail survival of the fittest. If you are no longer feeling sexually viable, one might postulate that it may be a stroke against your own evolutionary status. Maintaining healthy hormonal balance, managing stress, and ensuring good nutritional status are crucial for a healthy libido. Certain supplements may also correct sexual dysfunction, such as impotence or low sperm count, when taken properly.

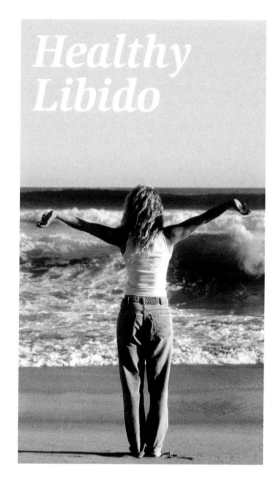

Healthy Libido

Certain supplements may correct sexual dysfunction, such as impotence or low sperm count, when taken properly.

Prevent Premature Aging

Thousands of studies have proven that specific vitamins and supplements may aid in preventing diseases associated with aging. For instance, calcium supplements can help to prevent osteoporosis, vitamin B-12 can help to prevent heart disease by lowering homocysteine levels, and selenium protects the prostate.

Guidelines for Buying Vitamins

Convinced yet? Clearly, it is very, very difficult to get all the nutrients we need from our diet, even if we eat organic foods, everyday. Still, some people resist taking vitamins because they find them too pricey, while others feel that vitamins just give us expensive urine. Indeed, if you are not careful about the products you are buying, this statement may be true.

Shopping for vitamins is a daunting task. Shelves in drugstores, health-food stores, and vitamin shops are lined with hundreds of products from scores of suppliers. New products and new research on these products appear daily — just keeping up-to-date is a full time job in itself. So, how do we know what vitamins and minerals to buy? What's a fair price? Here are some guidelines you can use in choosing good vitamins and minerals.

> "It's never too late to be what you might have been."
> George Elliot

Natural Is Better

Select the natural form of vitamins whenever possible. In general, natural forms of vitamins are better than synthetic forms. In some cases, synthetic vitamins cause health problems rather than prevent them. There are also fewer toxic reactions or potential intestinal upsets with natural forms. The natural forms may be slightly more expensive, but they are worth the investment.

Capsules vs. Tablets

Choose capsules, tablets, powders, and liquids that are highly absorbable. Some forms of vitamins and minerals are more readily absorbed than others. Capsules are usually more absorbable than tablets, but if the tablets are made by a reputable company, they can be just as absorbable as capsules, and, in some cases, they may be superior. Traditionally, tablets are broken down by stomach acids, but some companies make their tablets to dissolve at specific temperatures to ensure maximum absorption. However, some tablets and timed-released pills may be difficult to break down, particularly if you are experiencing low levels of stomach acid or digestive enzymes. Powders or liquids are often a great option, especially for kids — just add them to smoothies or juice.

THE GOOD, THE BAD, AND THE UGLY

Imagine you are in the supplement section of your local drugstore and you have found two vitamin E products with the same quantity of capsules in both bottles. One sells for $10 the other, for $30. Which should you buy? Before you decide, let's consider why there may be a difference in price.

1. Check the form of the vitamin.

   The cheaper vitamin E may be synthetic, not natural. Synthetic vitamin E is associated with side effects. You would want to buy the natural source vitamin in this case, despite the price difference.

2. Consider the dose.

   Perhaps the cheaper option is only 200 IU, not 400 IU or 800 IU, all common dosages.

3. Check the composition of the supplement.

   Maybe the cheaper vitamin E contains only one type of vitamin E, while the more expensive option contains all eight types of vitamin E. Taking a supplement containing only one type of vitamin E can result in a deficiency of the others, which are essential for protection against cancer.

As you can see through this example, if you go for the cheaper product, you are wasting your money and perhaps doing more harm than good. In this instance, the extra $20 is money well spent (or think of it as more savings in your health bank).

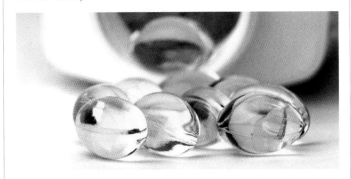

Chelation

Check labels for the words "citrate" or "chelate" to ensure you are taking the most absorbable form of multivitamin. Better multivitamins have their vitamins and minerals in highly absorbable forms, like amino acid chelates and citrates, rather than sulfates, carbonates, or oxides, although these less absorbable forms are still good for many purposes. Amino acid-bound, chelated mineral supplements can provide 3 to 10 times better assimilation than the non-chelated forms.

Check labels for the words "citrate" or "chelate" to ensure you are taking the most absorbable form of multivitamin.

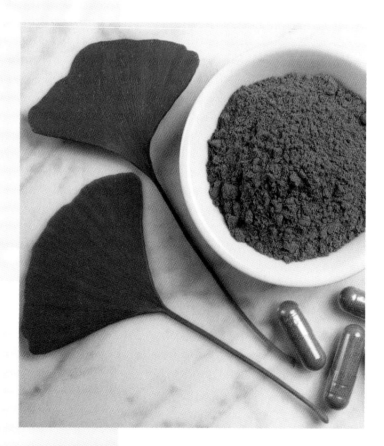

ODI vs. RDA

When comparing products, note their optimal daily intake or ODI rather than their recommended daily allowance or RDA. Be sure that the minimum ODI intake suggested for each vitamin is obtainable with a reasonable number of capsules or tablets per day.

The RDA represents the minimum level of the nutrient required to prevent deficiency diseases when one is otherwise in good health, while the ODI is the optimal level of the nutrient for therapeutic effect. Many people believe that much higher doses than the RDAs are beneficial, especially in the prevention of health problems, such as heart disease and cancer. Vitamins may also be taken in higher dosages for shorter periods of time for therapeutic effect. For example, vitamin C and zinc may be taken at higher levels during a cold or flu. Folic acid may be taken at doses of 5 mg per day or more to treat and prevent cervical dysplasia.

While health organizations have established official RDA tables, the ODI is an unofficial range of nutrient values designed to address optimal health and the prevention of disease based on clinical studies. The levels are similar to what a doctor would prescribe.

RECOMMENDED DAILY ALLOWANCE VS. OPTIMAL DAILY ALLOWANCE OF VITAMINS & MINERALS

Vitamins				Minerals		
Nutrient	RDA	ODI		Nutrient	RDA	ODI
Vitamin A	5,000 IU	5,000-10,000 IU		Boron	No RDA	3 mg
Beta-carotene	No RDA	10,000-25,000 IU		Calcium	1,000 mg	1,000-1,500 mg
Vitamin B-1	1.5 mg	25-300 mg		Copper	2 mg	0.5-2.5 mg
Vitamin B-2	1.7 mg	25-300 mg		Iodine	150 mcg	150-200 mcg
Vitamin B-3	20 mg	25-300 mg		Iron	Males: 10 mg	Males: 5-15 mg
Vitamin B-5	10 mg	25-500 mg			Females: 18 mg	Females: 18-30 mg
Vitamin B-6	2 mg	25-300 mg		Magnesium	400 mg	400-700 mg
Vitamin B-12	6 mcg	25-500 mcg		Manganese	2 mg	15-30 mg
Vitamin B-15	No RDA	25-100 mg		Phosphorus	400 mg	400-1,000 mg
Vitamin C	60 mg	500-2,000 mg		Potassium	99 mg	99 mg
Vitamin D	400 IU	400-800 IU		Selenium	70 mcg	50-200 mcg
Vitamin E	30 IU	400-800 IU		Zinc	15 mg	15-50 mg
Vitamin K	80 mcg	80 mcg				
Biotin	300 mcg	300 mcg				
Choline	No RDA	50-500 mg				
Folic Acid	400 mcg	400-1,200 mcg				
Inositol	No RDA	50-500 mg				
GABA	No RDA	50-500 mg				

Multivitamin Micronutrients

Consider the amounts of critical micronutrients needed to prevent specific health disorders, such as boron (bone disorders and arthritis) and vanadium (blood sugar and immune disorders). These are included in some vegetables and fruits, but you may need to supplement your diet with a multivitamin if you do not obtain enough in your food. The major vitamins and minerals, such as A, B, C, E and zinc, are usually more important for most people than these micronutrients, but they can be a useful measure for gauging the quality or suitability of a multivitamin.

Vitamin K Caution

Some individuals may require vitamin K for bone health or proper blood clotting, while others may need to avoid it. Patients on blood thinners (warfarin or Coumadin) or with heart disease should not take vitamin K or a multivitamin with vitamin K included.

Mixed Vitamin E

Since most multivitamins contain only the alpha tocopherol type of vitamin E, we recommend taking a mixed vitamin E product to make sure you have all your bases covered. There are eight types of tocopherols that make up vitamin E.

A form of vitamin E containing all eight types of tocopherols, not just alpha tocopherols, should be taken in conjunction with your multivitamin. Taking alpha tocopherols alone may cause a deficiency of the other seven types of tocopherols in the body. Tocopherols provide necessary antioxidant protection and promote cardiovascular health as we age.

Iron Limits

Most responsible health professionals recommend avoiding iron supplements unless a deficiency has been diagnosed. Men and postmenopausal women, in particular, should avoid supplements

A form of vitamin E containing all eight types of tocopherols, not just alpha tocopherols, should be taken in conjunction with your multivitamin.

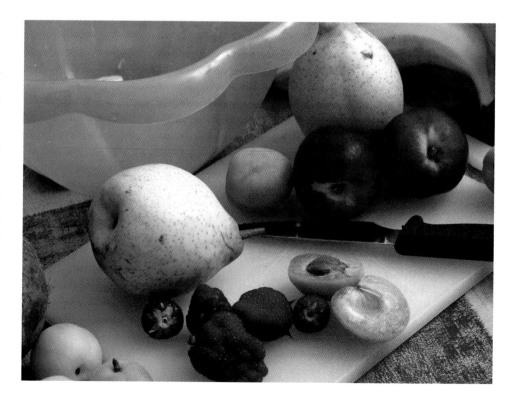

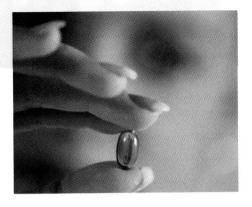

with iron. Most companies offer iron-free formulas of their multivitamins, or include just a small amount, in the 25% RDA range. Unless there are special needs, only children and pre-menopausal women should take supplements with a significant amount of iron.

Filler Free

Choose multivitamins and all other supplement products that are free of binders, fillers, artificial colorings, preservatives, yeast, sugar, starch, or other additives. Most people who have reactions to vitamins tend to have issues with the additives.

Herbal Remedies

When purchasing an herbal remedy, such as valerian or echinacea, be sure the label says it is "standardized." If a product is standardized, it means it is guaranteed to contain a certain amount of active ingredient. There is a big difference between taking 500 mg of an herb that is not standardized and 500 mg of an herb that is guaranteed to contain 45% of the active ingredient. Or between purchasing the root of a plant when it is the leaf that contains the active constituents for medicinal effect.

GOOD RESOURCES

Be aware of your options when selecting vitamins and be sure you know what you are looking for. For more information, we suggest consulting a book called the *Comparative Guide to Nutritional Supplements*, which provides an independent, third-party analysis of all of the multivitamins available in North America. This guide rates the quality of a multivitamin based upon ingredients, dosage, and absorption. In general, any product with a score greater than 70 is a suitable choice, but the closer the score to 100, the better the product. Use this guide to check the vitamins you are taking now. You may be surprised at the money and effort you have been wasting.

When purchasing an herbal remedy, such as valerian or echinacea, be sure the label says that it is "standardized."

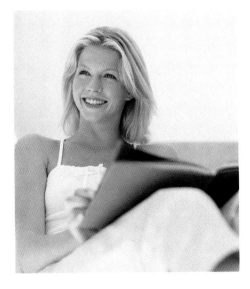

Truestar Health Professional Series of Vitamins

Following these basic guidelines requires knowing a great deal about the composition, preparation, packaging, and action of any given vitamin and mineral. This level of detail is more than most people can manage alone. Many people simply don't have the time to go to 'vitamin' school. They look for a reliable brand that provides the best nutrients, at a fair price, without having to worry about dosage dangers and side effects.

The Truestar Health Professional Series product line offers premium, professional-strength supplements that assure maximum absorption and potency. These doctor-prescribed, clinically-tested, effective formulas have previously been available only through physicians and pharmacists, but are now available directly to you online at www.truestarhealth.com and at Truestar for Women Health & Fitness Centers.

The Truestar vitamin line contains products at therapeutic doses, which distinguishes them from many of the best-selling vitamins available in pharmacies and health-food stores. The Truestar Health Professional Series is formulated with consideration of the ODI and can be used for therapeutic effect because of the potency of our products.

It is our priority to stay on the cutting edge of nutritional supplements and to be leaders in our field while ensuring you receive the best products for health promotion at any age.

TrueBASICS

Let's look, for example, at TrueBASICS, our enhanced multivitamin pack, to see how the qualities we have specified for good vitamins are met — and even surpassed.

> Many people simply don't have the time to go to 'vitamin' school. They look for a reliable brand that provides the best nutrients, at a fair price, without having to worry about dosage dangers and side effects.

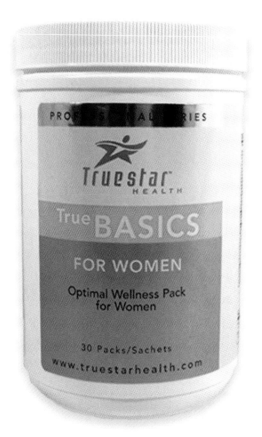

Log on to www.truestarhealth.com to create a personal vitamin plan based on your weight-loss goals, physical activity level, and current health status.

TrueBASICS contains five ingredients prepared in the most absorbable and beneficial forms for your health.

1. Calcium — Magnesium with Vitamin D-3 tablets
2. Mixed Vitamin E capsule
3. Grapeseed Extract tablet
4. Fish Oil capsule
5. Multivitamin tablets

CAL-MAG:

Case in point, our calcium-magnesium is prepared in the most absorbable citrate form, rather than in calcium carbonate form. A National Institutes of Health (NIH) study showed that calcium supplementation slowed bone loss (osteoporosis) and decreased the number of bone fractures. Our cal-mag supplement also includes vitamin D-3, which is best for bones, rather than D-2.

MIXED VITAMIN E:

We use high-quality, natural, mixed vitamin E in TrueBASICS. This does raise the price, but we believe your health is worth the investment. We include seven times more vitamin E than our competitors do. A study conducted at Harvard University and published in *The New England Journal of Medicine* found that vitamin E reduced the risk of coronary heart disease in both men and women.

GRAPE SEED EXTRACT:

Grape seed extract is a strong antioxidant that helps maintain blood vessels. Our competitors do not include this in their preparations.

FISH OIL:

We provide essential fatty acid (EFA) fish oils containing both EPA and DHA in the TrueBASICS pack, while our competitors do not.

MULTIVITAMIN:

The multivitamin is highly potent pharmaceutical grade, with all ingredients in the most absorbable forms. We include micronutrients and greater ODI quantities than our competitors.

- VITAMIN C: We include four to five times more vitamin C than our competitors. Studies have shown that vitamin C reduces the risk of cataracts, enhances the immune system, and reduces the risk of heart attacks.
- IRON: Our men's pack is iron free because men normally do not need iron, while women do because they tend to lose iron monthly until menopause.
- CALCIUM: Our basic multivitamin for women over 45 contains nutrients specific for bones strength and mass, as well as more calcium.
- MAGNESIUM: Magnesium has been shown to lower blood pressure and increase bone density in people with osteoporosis. We include eight times more magnesium than our competitors do.
- N-ACETYL CYSTEINE (NAC): NAC is a potent antioxidant and a liver-supporting supplement. Our competitors do not include it in their basic multivitamin.

Log on to www.truestarhealth.com for a guide to the full line of Truestar Health Professional Series supplements.

Other Truestar Vitamins

Phew… so many issues were considered when the TrueBASICS pack was formulated. The same amount of work went into developing each product in the Truestar Health Professional Series. We offer superior quality, innovative products, and the highest possible vitamin quantities, while maintaining a competitive price.

The Truestar Health Professional Series of vitamins and supplements is made by one of the leading nutritional laboratories in North America. We demand superior quality materials throughout every step of the manufacturing process. Our vitamins and supplements are made according to strict, meticulously-followed quality control standards. Our products are stringently sampled and tested before they are released to our consumers. All products in the Truestar Health Professional Series are made in compliance with the Good Manufacturing Practices (GMPs).

The Truestar Health Professional Series also offers cutting-edge nutritional supplements based on the latest scientific research. For example, our heart health product, TrueCARDIO, contains coenzyme Q10, a supplement recently proven to increase the effectiveness of the heart. Our weight loss product, TrueLEAN, contains conjugated linoleic acid (CLA), found to reduce abdominal obesity.

For a guide to the full line of Truestar Health Professional Series supplements, log on at www.truestarhealth.com.

All products in the Truestar Health Professional Series are made in compliance with the Good Manufacturing Practices (GMPs).

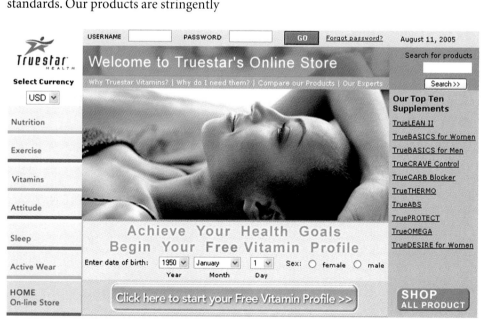

Truestar Vitamin Programs

At Truestar, we create individualized vitamin programs using our vitamin profiling system online at www.truestarhealth.com. You can also use our vitamin plan chart reproduced here to develop your own vitamin regimen.

Vitamin Profile Program

At www.truestarhealth.com, your personal vitamin prescription is formulated through your answers to our vitamin profile questions. You can determine your vitamin plan by means of a comprehensive health and lifestyle analysis or via a particular health goal. If you choose by a current health goal, a group of products that work synergistically to address your particular concern, such as weight loss, healthy skin, or joint health, is provided specific to age and sex. This is unique to the Truestar supplement program and makes our vitamin profiling system as close as you can get to naturopathic treatment, without a one-on-one office visit.

When you complete our online health history and lifestyle vitamin profile, you may find several products are recommended for you. It is best to begin with the 'foundation' products. When multiple products appear in the highly recommended and beneficial categories, determine which products you would like to add to your plan by clicking "Why

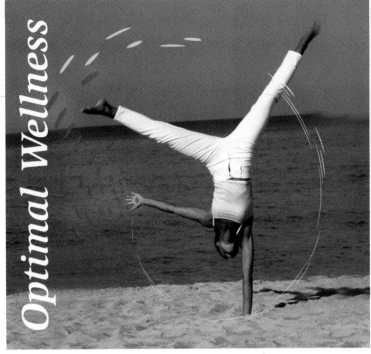

Optimal Wellness

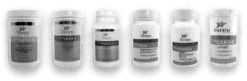

- TrueBASICS For Women
- TrueLEAN 3
- TruePROTECT
- TrueCELL
- TrueOMEGA
- TrueCARDIO Support

Choose This?" next to each product listed. This allows you to determine the primary mode of action/benefit of each product. You can use this information to chose specific supplements that focus upon your greatest concerns. Remember, your profile results are saved and can be viewed at any time by clicking "vitamins view plan" on the "my plans" page.

Regardless of the method you choose to create your vitamin plan, our system provides recommendations based upon the latest clinical research and the most up-to-date discoveries for health promotion and preventive medicine.

Our vitamin profiling system is as close as you can get to naturopathic treatment, without a one-on-one office visit.

Weight-Loss Supplement Plan

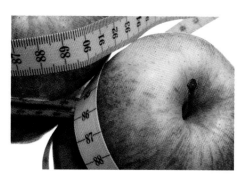

Let's look at how your vitamin program can be customized to promote weight loss through the three phases described in the Nutrition chapter — the Metabolic Booster Plan, the Weight-Loss Continuum Plan, and the Weight-Loss Maintenance Plan.

The quest for the perfect body is never ending and many will adopt whatever means necessary to achieve it. No doubt, exercise and proper diet are essential for a healthy body composition, but what about weight-loss aids? Most products marketed for weight loss have little research to support their claims, but there are a few select products that do work to increase fat burning and to boost metabolism when used properly. It is these supplements, supported with clinical results, that form the basis of our vitamin weight-loss program.

Sad to say, I do not think for one second that weight loss comes solely from a bottle. Albeit, significant research does show the benefit of certain products used

The secret to weight loss comes in a bottle? Ah, if only life were that sweet …

in conjunction with a weight-loss plan. Through studying this research and compiling results, we have developed a supplement program uniquely designed to complement our phase-based nutrition plan. This vitamin program enhances your nutritional and exercise programs by detoxifying your body, conquering food cravings, stimulating metabolism, and optimizing your energy.

The secret to weight loss comes in a bottle? Ah, if only life were that sweet …

PHASE I

Metabolic Booster Phase Supplements

TrueBASICS

This pack should be taken during all phases of your Truestar weight-loss program. But why is BASICS so necessary for use during weight loss when it does not contain the ingredients typical of a weight-loss aid?

- BASICS contains calcium proven to assist weight loss. This is the reason why dairy products are currently being touted as one of the best foods for weight loss.
- BASICS provides several antioxidants, such as grape seed extract and vitamin C, that offer protection during the process of weight loss when fat cells release a lot of waste and stored 'junk' as they are broken down.

- BASICS prevents vitamin deficiency. A deficiency of just one nutrient can slow metabolism. For example, a deficiency of zinc, selenium, or B vitamins can decrease the production of thyroid hormone, which governs our metabolism.
- BASICS decreases cravings. A deficiency of chromium or magnesium can result in increased cravings for sugar and chocolate.
- BASICS replenishes our store of nutrients and combats free radicals. We naturally require more nutrients and antioxidants when we exercise because it stimulates our metabolism and therefore increases the production of waste products in the body. Antioxidants help to combat the harmful effects of these compounds, referred to as free radicals.
- BASICS provides extra vitamin E, proven to reduce muscle stiffness and soreness after exercise.
- BASICS provides extra calcium and magnesium daily, which help proper muscle contraction and relaxation, as well as fish oils, which assist with the prevention of joint pain and stiffness and have been proven to encourage fat loss.

> Fish oils assist with the prevention of joint pain and stiffness and have been proven to encourage fat loss.

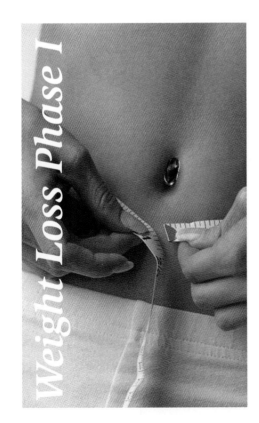

Weight Loss Phase I

TrueLEAN III

Your weight-loss plan begins with our detoxification and weight-loss support product, TrueLEAN III. Taking TrueLEAN III for the first 4 to 6 weeks will cleanse the bowel and liver. TrueLEAN III helps to combat constipation associated with the restriction of grains in your Phase I diet because it contains two fiber capsules and an herbal formula to increase the flow of bile. Also contained in this pack are two herbs to boost thyroid function (which stimulates our metabolism) and a natural diuretic formula to reduce water retention and bloating. For optimal results, take one pack 15 to 30 minutes before meals twice a day. This product is ideal for the first 4 to 6 weeks, but can be continued for the duration of the weight-loss program, if you so desire.

TrueCRAVING Control

With the restriction of sugar and starch in Phase I, we naturally tend to have increased cravings for these satisfying 'comfort' foods. To help you resist these cravings and stress-related eating patterns, we recommend taking True-CRAVING Control for the first 2 to 3 weeks. Complete with chromium, glutamine, magnesium, 5 HTP, and many other ingredients, this product works well for cravings if taken at the full dose. You may begin taking TrueCRAVING Control a few days or a week prior to starting Phase I of your weight loss plan if you feel you are really hooked on carbs.

TrueTHERMO

You can give your metabolism an even greater boost with our thermogenic aid, TrueTHERMO taken in conjunction with TrueCRAVE and TrueLEAN III. TrueTHERMO contains a mixture of herbal products that increase fat burning and boost metabolism. It should not be taken by individuals who have high blood pressure, heart disease, epilepsy, or a history of heart attack or stroke because it does have an action like caffeine. TrueTHERMO contains green tea and tyrosine, two ingredients proven to assist the body during carbohydrate restriction, to support thyroid function,

TrueTHERMO contains green tea and tyrosine, two ingredients proven to assist the body during carbohydrate restriction, to support thyroid function, to boost fat loss, and to control appetite.

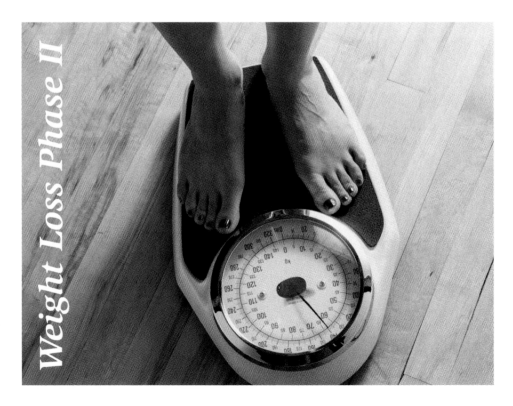

Weight Loss Phase II

to boost fat loss, and to control appetite. It is best to take this product at a dose of 1 to 2 pills per day, particularly before a workout and not too late in the day.

TrueSTRENGTH

We recommend whey protein powder for our smoothies because studies show whey protein, more so than other protein types, encourages a greater loss of body fat.

PHASE II

Continuum Weight-Loss Phase Supplements

TrueCRAVING Control

Unless you are still experiencing carbohydrate carvings, it is not necessary to continue the use of TrueCRAVING Control.

TrueLEAN II

In Phase II, when your detox is completed, we recommend taking TrueLEAN II, but if you experience constipation, water retention, or you wish to continue the use of guggulipids and coleus forskholin to stimulate metabolism, you can continue taking TrueLEAN III along with TrueLEAN II. TrueLEAN II contains conjugated linoleic acid and green tea. Both ingredients have been proven to encourage weight loss. Green tea results in fat loss without a change in diet or exercise (not that we ever recommend it!). TrueLEAN II also contains a weight-loss formula containing chromium and hydroxycitric acid that

control appetite and regulate blood sugar levels.

TrueCARB BLOCKER

In this phase of your weight-loss plan, you will add modest amounts of carbohydrates back into your diet. To reduce the risk of weight gain, we recommend the use of TrueCARB BLOCKER prior to your meal of the day that contains starch. When taken correctly, TrueCARB BLOCKER may reduce the absorption of starches and fats, thereby assisting with weight loss. It's also great for parties or special dinners out. This product maintains lower blood sugar levels after eating. As a result, less insulin is released in response to the meal, which is always good for weight reduction.

TrueTHERMO

You can continue to give your metabolism maximum support with TrueTHERMO.

PHASE III

Weight-Loss Maintenance Phase Supplements

In this phase, you have two options. You may continue taking TrueLEAN II at the maintenance dose of one pack per day, taking our other weight-loss formulas as necessary. Or you may complete our vitamin profile online at www.truestarhealth.com or select from any one of the vitamin plans on the Vitamin Plan Chart to determine the best products for your optimal health and wellness.

To reduce the risk of weight gain, we recommend taking TrueCARB BLOCKER prior to your meal of the day that contains starch.

Vitamin Plan Chart

You can use this quick reference chart we have provided to help you create a daily vitamin plan that addresses your specific health concerns and maintains ongoing good health.

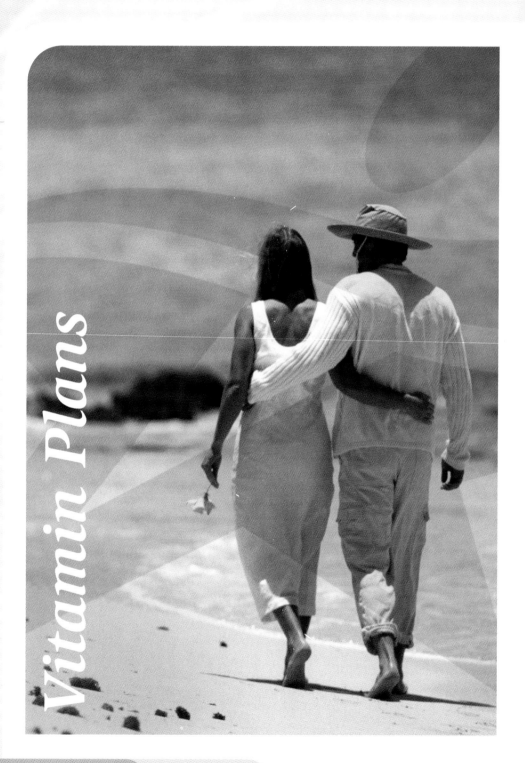

Vitamin Plans

PRODUCT	RATING	WHY CHOOSE
ADD/ADHD		
TrueBASICS	●	Studies show proper nutrition and supplementation with essential nutrients are important for concentration, cognition, and learning. TrueBASICS contains the ingredients necessary for basic support for all ages.
TrueOMEGA Enteric-coated soft gels for cardiovascular health, brain health, and wellness	●	TrueOMEGA contains a pharmaceutical grade DHA concentrated fish oil. DHA can improve learning and memory. It is an important structural component of the brain and nervous system.
TruePROTECT Basic Antioxidant Support	●	TruePROTECT contains zinc and magnesium — both have been found to improve the symptoms of ADD/ADHD. Zinc is found in the brain's hippocampus and interacts with other chemicals to send messages to the sensory brain center, enhancing memory and thinking skills. It has a significant effect on visual memory, learning, emotional and behavioral states, and overall cognitive function. Magnesium supplements can promote relaxation, focus, attention and restful sleep.
ALLERGIES		
TrueBASICS	●	TrueBASICS contains the building blocks of a healthy immune system. Taken daily, this product helps to prevent nutrient deficiency, which may weaken the immune system and increase the risk of infections or colds and flus.
TrueALLERFREE Quercetin-Bromelain complex	●	TrueALLERFREE contains quercetin and bromelain for the treatment of allergies, free of the side effects commonly associated with OTC antihistamines.
TrueC	●	Vitamin C, a natural antihistamine, is essential for a healthy immune system and can support your body through the stress of allergies.
TrueDOPHILUS Beneficial flora for healthy intestinal function	●	Acidophilus supplements may aid allergic symptoms because of the close association between the digestive tract and the immune system — 60% of our immune system surrounds the digestive tract.

PRODUCT	RATING	WHY CHOOSE
ANTI-AGING		
TrueBASICS	●	TrueBASICS contains grapeseed extract and a mixed vitamin E — potent antioxidants that are very protective to the heart, brain and skin cells.
TruePROTECT Basic antioxidant support	●	Taking antioxidants, such as vitamin C, E, and A, zinc, and selenium, protects our cells from aging due to free radical damage. TruePROTECT assists with keeping our skin looking younger, our brain sharper, our eyes clearer, and our heart healthier.
TrueCELL Coenzyme Q10 with lipoic acid	●	TrueCELL contains two potent anti-aging compounds, alpha lipoic acid (ALA) and coenzyme Q10, helping to reduce the risk of wrinkles and age spots.
TrueSIGHT Eye health support with Lutein	●	TrueSight contains lutein to protect the eye from macular degeneration and the effects of aging due to its natural antioxidant properties.
TrueIQ Brain and nervous system protector with acetyl-L-carnitine	●	Acetyl-L-carnitine is a potent anti-aging compound for the brain, which may assist in maintaining memory and preventing Alzheimer's disease.
AUTOIMMUNE DISEASE		
TrueBASICS	●	TrueBASICS contains the building blocks of a healthy immune system. Taken daily, this product helps to prevent nutrient deficiency, which may weaken the immune system and increase the risk of infections or colds and flus. It also aids the body during times of physical stress like in autoimmune disease. In autoimmune disease, the immune system is constantly active. It is one of the most energetically expensive systems in the body — don't leave yourself lacking in nutrients!
TrueMODULATE Immune modulating with plant sterol complex	●	TrueMODULATE contains plant sterols useful in autoimmune diseases, such as rheumatoid arthritis, by helping to slow down an overactive immune system.

PRODUCT	RATING	WHY CHOOSE
DIABETES AND HEALTHY BLOOD SUGAR BALANCE		
TrueBASICS	●	TrueBASICS contains fish oils known to improve body composition and insulin sensitivity. The vitamin E and grapeseed extract help to protect the eyes, brain, heart, and blood vessels — all at risk with blood sugar diseases.
TrueCONTROL nutritional support for healthy blood sugar balance	●	Healthy blood sugar balance is crucial for optimal energy levels, weight management, reduction of the risk of type II diabetes, cholesterol levels, and stress hormone balance.
TrueABS Healthy insulin response and body composition support with conjugated linoleic acid and green tea	●	Because of its effects on insulin response, conjugated linoleic acid (CLA) may aid symptoms of hypoglycemia and blood sugar balance.
TrueCARB Blocker	●	TrueCARB Blocker taken once a day with meals containing starch and fat may help to maintain healthy blood sugar balance.
ENDURANCE ATHLETES		
TrueBASICS	●	Exercise elevates your nutrient needs as sweating increases nutrient loss, including B vitamins and zinc, and the subsequent boost in metabolism increases our need for antioxidants. Vitamin E can aid recovery after exercise, and calcium-magnesium is crucial for proper muscle growth, contraction, and relaxation. Do not leave your body lacking for vitamins, minerals, and antioxidants by missing your BASICS daily. Your performance may suffer!
TrueSUPPORT Botanical blend for healthy mental support and stress reduction with relora and vitamin B complex	●	Training for endurance sports is a physical stress on the body. Relora, the herbal blend contained in TrueSUPPORT, helps to keep the body strong, healthy, and resilient during training by preventing abnormal elevations of stress hormones that can suppress the immune system and damage muscle fibers.
TruePROTECT Basic antioxidant support	●	Exercise increases the need for extra antioxidant protection. Vitamins E and C in this product may also help to reduce soreness after exercise.

PRODUCT	RATING	WHY CHOOSE
TrueSTRENGTH Whey protein powder	●	Whey protein assists with lean muscle mass, aids recovery from exercise, maintains a healthy immune system, helps prevent the symptoms of over-training, and aids with weight loss.
EYE HEALTH		
TrueBASICS	●	TrueBASICS contains the nutrients necessary for a healthy immune system, high energy levels, and nutrient-deficiency prevention. The mixed vitamin E, fish oils, and grapeseed extract in this formula are important for protection of the eye from free radicals involved in the formation of cataracts and may assist dry eye syndrome.
TrueSIGHT Eye health support with lutein	●	Lutein is a potent antioxidant for the eyes and protects them from damage.
TrueOMEGA Enteric-coated soft gels for cardiovascular health, brain health, and wellness	●	DHA fish oils are building blocks for the eyes and nervous system. Taking fish oils daily can help combat dry eyes and maintain ocular health.
TruePROTECT Basic antioxidant support	●	The vitamins C, E, A and zinc in TruePROTECT guard the eyes from oxidative damage and are useful in the treatment and prevention of cataracts.
FATIGUE		
TrueBASICS	●	A deficiency of just one nutrient is enough to cause fatigue. Do not leave yourself lacking! Drinking coffee, taking medications, and even exercise increases your nutrient needs. The B vitamins, magnesium, zinc, and vitamin C in this formula are crucial to maintaining and improving your energy levels throughout the day.
TrueB Formula High potency B-complex	●	Supplements of B vitamins may assist with fatigue and energy levels.
TrueSUPPORT Botanical blend for healthy mental support and stress reduction with relora and vitamin B complex	●	TrueSUPPORT contains the herbal blend relora, which assists the body during times of stress and helps prevent burnout.

PRODUCT	RATING	WHY CHOOSE
TrueADAPT Ashwaganda stress support	◐	Ashwaganda, the herb contained in TrueADAPT, is unique in that it can be both stress-supporting and energy-boosting.
TrueTHERMO	◐	TrueTHERMO contains green tea, tyrosine, and other herbs that have energy-boosting and metabolism-enhancing properties. This product is great for a quick pick-me-up, especially before a workout.
HEALTHY DIGESTION		
TrueBASICS	●	TrueBASICS contains ingredients necessary for a healthy immune system, high energy levels, and nutrient-deficiency prevention. If you have a digestive condition, your nutrient absorption could be compromised. TrueBASICS ensures you have the foundation of health.
TrueDIGEST Comprehensive digestive enzyme support	●	Digestive enzymes are particularly useful to reduce gas, and bloating or bowel irregularities associated with IBS. They may also reduce the symptoms associated with food allergies and assist with nutrient absorption.
TrueDOPHILUS Beneficial flora for healthy intestinal function	●	Acidophilus supplements aid bacterial balance necessary for healthy digestion and absorption.
TrueADAPT Ashwaganda stress support	◐	Ashwaganda is unique in that it can be both stress-supporting and energy-boosting. It is useful for anxiety because it increases the production of calming hormones. There is a well-documented connection between stress and irritable bowel syndrome.
TrueSOOTHE Digestive healing and immunity support with DGL	◐	TrueSOOTHE contains DGL, a type of licorice which can coat and heal the digestive tract. It is excellent for reducing symptoms of heartburn, reflux, ulcers, and indigestion. This product is useful in conjunction with medications used for Gastro Esophagel Reflex Disease (GERD) or heartburn because it helps reduce symptoms, as well as repair the damage or irritation in the gut. Most medications for these conditions focus only on symptomatic relief. DGL also aids inflammatory bowel conditions, such as Crohn's disease or ulcerative colitis.

PRODUCT	RATING	WHY CHOOSE
TrueBuild Glutamine 500 mg capsules with Gastro-intestinal support	●	Glutamine is very effective in the treatment of diarrhea and helps to repair the cells of the digestive tract wall.

HEALTHY IMMUNITY

PRODUCT	RATING	WHY CHOOSE
TrueBASICS for Women 45+ and Bone Health Optimal wellness pack	●	TrueBASICS contains ingredients necessary for a healthy immune system, high energy levels, and nutrient deficiency prevention. TrueBASICS ensures you have the foundation of health, and the vitamin A, C, E, and zinc in this pack help to keep your immune system strong!
TrueC Antioxidant and immune support with 1000 mg ascorbic acid	●	Vitamin C is essential for a healthy immune system. Vitamin C should be taken daily for cold and flu prevention. The dose can be increased if you are currently experiencing signs of an infection.
TrueDEFENSE Immune support formula	●	TrueDEFENSE contains a combination of immune-enhancing herbs, such as astragalus, echinacea, ginseng, and garlic, and the mineral zinc to improve your natural defenses. This product can be used at a low dose, as needed, to prevent a cold or flu, or at a higher dose to treat symptoms of an existing infection.
TrueDOPHILUS Beneficial flora for healthy intestinal function	●	Supplements of acidophilus may reduce allergic symptoms or prevent their onset, decrease the frequency of colds and the flu, and assist with better recovery time from illness and surgery.

HEALTHY JOINTS

PRODUCT	RATING	WHY CHOOSE
TrueBASICS	●	TrueBASICS contains ingredients necessary for a healthy immune system, high energy levels, and nutrient-deficiency prevention. TrueBASICS ensures the foundation of health. In this formula, the calcium-magnesium is important for joint health, and the fish oil can reduce inflammation and joint pain.
TrueMSM Collagen and joint support with methylsulfonylmethane	●	MSM is a natural anti-inflammatory compound that contains sulfur, necessary for building and maintaining healthy joints.

PRODUCT	RATING	WHY CHOOSE
TrueRELIEF Botanical extracts to help reduce inflammation	●	TrueRELIEF contains tumeric, boswellia, and devil's claw, potent natural anti-inflammatory herbs that do not cause digestive irritation like aspirin and ibruprofen.
TrueMODULATE Immune modulating with plant sterol complex	●	TrueMODULATE contains plant sterols useful in autoimmune diseases, such as rheumatoid arthritis, by helping to slow down an overactive immune system.
TrueOMEGA Enteric-coated soft gels for cardiovascular health, brain health and wellness	●	Fish oils are natural anti-inflammatory compounds that can reduce pain and stiffness.
HEALTHY LIBIDO FOR MEN		
TrueBASICS	●	TrueBASICS contains ingredients necessary for a healthy immune system, high energy levels, and nutrient-deficiency prevention. TrueBASICS ensures the foundation of health. A healthy libido is an indication of your wellness — keep your mojo going with TrueBASICS.
TrueFLOW Heart and healthy circulation support with L-Arginine capsules	●	L-Arginine assists with increasing blood flow to the penis, aiding erectile dystunction (ED) related to circulatory causes.
TrueSUPPORT Botanical blend for healthy mental support and stress reduction with relora and vitamin B complex	●	High levels of stress hormone are linked to a low libido. TrueSUPPORT contains the herbal blend called relora, found to decrease the stress hormone cortisol and increase DHEA, the hormone important for a healthy libido and body composition.
HEALTHY LIBIDO FOR WOMEN		
TrueBASICS	●	TrueBASICS contains ingredients necessary for a healthy immune system, high energy levels, and nutrient-deficiency prevention. TrueBASICS ensures the foundation of health. A healthy libido is an indication of your health — keep your mojo going with TrueBASICS.

● Highly Recommended
● Beneficial

PRODUCT	RATING	WHY CHOOSE
TrueDESIRE for Women Libido-boost formula	●	A healthy libido is a sign of good health. If you have noticed a change in your libido, it may be an indication that something is out of balance. Regular use of TrueDESIRE may assist with restoring a healthy libido.
TrueSUPPORT Botanical blend for healthy mental support and stress reduction with relora and vitamin B complex	●	High levels of stress hormone are linked to a low libido. TrueSUPPORT contains relora, found to decrease the stress hormone cortisol and increase DHEA, the hormone important for a healthy libido and body composition.
TrueMENO Comprehensive nutritional support during menopause	●	TrueMENO contains herbal ingredients that assist with symptoms associated with changing levels of estrogen and progesterone in menopause that can affect libido. TrueMENO may offer a replacement to synthetic HRT with the advice of your doctor.

HEALTHY MIND AND MEMORY

TrueBASICS	●	TrueBASICS contains ingredients necessary for a healthy immune system, high energy levels, and nutrient-deficiency prevention. TrueBASICS ensures the foundation of health. Taking vitamin C and vitamin E daily can reduce your risk of Alzheimer's disease by 58%! The fish oil and the grapeseed extract in this formula protect brain cells and cognitive function.
TrueOMEGA Enteric-coated soft gels for cardiovascular health, brain health, and wellness	●	DHA fish oils are building blocks of the brain and nervous system. They protect the brain from harmful amounts of stress hormones that naturally tend to increase as we age. Supplements of fish oil may improve memory and cognitive function in aging populations.
TrueIQ Brain and nervous system protector with Acetyl-L-carnitine	●	Acetyl-L-carnitine is a potent anti-aging compound for the brain that may assist with maintaining memory and preventing Alzheimer's disease.

PRODUCT	RATING	WHY CHOOSE
TrueCARE Essential nutrients to support homocysteine metabolism	●	High levels of homocysteine (>7) increase the risk of Alzheimer's disease. Homocysteine may also be elevated in cases of depression and memory loss. TrueCARE, taken daily, can reduce homocysteine, and the risk of Alzheimer's disease, as well as improve cognitive function.
TrueMEMORY Support for healthy mental and circulatory function with Ginkgo biloba capsules	●	TrueMEMORY contains Ginkgo, which can increase circulation to the brain and assist with memory and recall, particularly in older individuals.
TrueSUPPORT Botanical blend for healthy mental support and stress reduction with relora and vitamin B complex.	●	High levels of stress hormone are linked to memory loss and damage to the area of the brain involved in memory. TrueSUPPORT contains relora, which works by decreasing the stress hormone cortisol, thereby protecting brain cells. Relora also increases DHEA, the hormone important for healthy libido, body composition, and mental function.
HEALTHY PROSTATE		
TrueBASICS	●	TrueBASICS contains ingredients necessary for a healthy immune system, high energy levels, and nutrient-deficiency prevention. TrueBASICS ensures the foundation of health. For the prostate in particular, the vitamin E, zinc, selenium, B vitamins, and vitamin A in this formula are all very beneficial.
TruePROSTATE Nutritional support for prostate health	●	TruePROSTATE is a combination of vitamins, minerals, amino acids, nutrients, and herbs, such as saw palmetto, *Pygeum africanum* and pumpkin seeds, designed to support prostate health and to prevent enlargement.
TruePROTECT Basic antioxidant support	●	TruePROTECT contains a blend of 6 vitamins and minerals that function as antioxidants in the body, thereby aiding and maintaining cellular health. Antioxidants are very important for cancer protection. Zinc and the selenium contained in TruePROTECT are protective to prostate gland cells.

PRODUCT	RATING	WHY CHOOSE
HEALTHY SKIN		
TrueBASICS	●	TrueBASICS contains ingredients necessary for a healthy immune system, high energy levels, and nutrient-deficiency prevention. TrueBASICS ensures the foundation of health. For the skin in particular, the grapeseed, vitamin E, zinc, selenium, B vitamins, and vitamin A in this formula are beneficial. The fish oils and mixed vitamin E moisturize from the inside out!
TruePROTECT Basic antioxidant support	●	TruePROTECT contains vitamins C, A and E, as well as zinc, essential to healthy skin, healing, and collagen formation.
TrueOMEGA Enteric-coated soft gels for cardiovascular health, brain health, and wellness	●	Essential fatty acids can moisten the skin, reduce itching, treat and prevent eczema, and prevent wrinkling because of their natural anti-inflammatory and moisturizing properties.
TrueDIGEST Comprehensive digestive enzyme support	●	If you have *Acne rosacea* (AR), this is an excellent addition to the skin plan. AR is often associated with a deficiency of hydrochloric acid and digestive enzymes. Taking this product can improve the condition of your skin and the absorption of your vitamins and minerals.
TrueMSM Collagen and joint support with Methylsulfonylmethane	●	MSM is a natural anti-inflammatory compound that contains sulfur, necessary for building and maintaining collagen in the skin.
HEART HEALTH		
TrueBASICS	●	TrueBASICS contains a fish oil, vitamin E, vitamin C, and grapeseed extract, proven to promote heart health. The calcium-magnesium combination assists with healthy blood pressure regulation and the multivitamin contains B vitamins, important for the reduction of homocysteine, an independent risk factor for heart disease.

PRODUCT	RATING	WHY CHOOSE
TrueOMEGA Enteric-coated soft gels for cardiovascular health, brain health, and wellness	◍	Hundreds of studies show that fish oils have cardio-protective qualities. Supplements can reduce cholesterol and blood pressure, assist with the maintenance of a healthy heart rhythm, and improve cardiac conditions, such as angina, heart attack, and stroke. For cardiovascular disease treatment and prevention, 4 g of fish oils should be taken daily. Remember, there is only 1 g in TrueBASICS.
TrueCARDIO Healthy heart pack	◍	TrueCARDIO contains nutrients that have beneficial effects on cholesterol levels, blood pressure, and homocysteine, as well as many other aspects of cardiovascular wellness.
TrueFLOW Heart and healthy circulation support with L-Arginine capsules	◍	TrueFLOW contains arginine, which provides antioxidant protection to the blood vessels and assists with healthy blood flow. It is useful in preventing arterial blockages and in lowering blood pressure.

HIGH BLOOD PRESSURE

PRODUCT	RATING	WHY CHOOSE
TrueBASICS	◍	TrueBASICS contains a fish oil, vitamin E, vitamin C, and grapeseed extract, proven to promote heart health. The calcium-magnesium combination assists with healthy blood pressure regulation. The multivitamin contains B vitamins, important for the reduction of homocysteine, an independent risk factor for heart disease.
TrueCARDIO Healthy heart pack	◍	TrueCARDIO contains hawthorne, which has beneficial effects on blood pressure regulation, as well as many other nutrients to assist with cardiovascular wellness.
TrueFLOW Heart and healthy circulation support with L-Arginine capsules	◍	L-Arginine in TrueFLOW has beneficial effects on blood pressure regulation through the production of nitric oxide.
TrueZZZs Melatonin	◍	Melatonin may be beneficial for high blood pressure. This product is better suited for individuals over 45 years of age.

PRODUCT	RATING	WHY CHOOSE
HIGH CHOLESTEROL		
TrueBASICS	●	TrueBASICS contains a fish oil, vitamin E, vitamin C, and grape-seed extract, proven to promote heart health. The calcium-magnesium combination assists with healthy blood pressure regulation, and the multivitamin contains B vitamins important for the reduction of homocysteine, an independent risk factor for heart disease.
TrueCARDIO Healthy heart pack	●	TrueCARDIO contains garlic, which has beneficial effects on cholesterol levels, as well as many other nutrients to assist with cardiovascular wellness.
TrueREDUCE Cholesterol-lowering formula	●	TrueREDUCE contains a blend of policosanols, red rice yeast extract, folic acid, and vitamin B-3 for effective reduction of elevated cholesterol levels.
TrueLEAN III	●	TrueLEAN III helps reduce elevated cholesterol levels. It contains 1 capsule of the herb called guggulipids and 2 fiber capsules. The liver-cleansing formula in this pack may help to prevent a fatty liver and assist the liver in healthy cholesterol metabolism.
TrueOMEGA Enteric-coated soft gels for cardiovascular health, brain health, and wellness	●	Hundreds of studies show the cardio-protective qualities of fish oils. Supplements can reduce cholesterol and blood pressure, assist with the maintenance of a healthy heart rhythm, and improve cardiac conditions, such as angina, heart attack, and stroke. For cardiovascular disease treatment and prevention, 4 g of fish oils should be taken daily. Remember, there is only 1 g in TrueBASICS.
HYPOTHYROIDISM		
TrueLEAN III	●	TrueLEAN III contains two herbs (guggulipids and coleus) shown to benefit thyroid gland function by increasing the production of the active form of thyroid hormone in the body that stimulates metabolism. This product is safe to take with thyroid medications, but should be taken at least 2 hours apart from other medication.

● Highly Recommended
● Beneficial

PRODUCT	RATING	WHY CHOOSE
TrueBASICS	●	Selenium, zinc, magnesium, essential fatty acids, vitamin A, and B complex are necessary for the proper formation of thyroid hormone in the body. TrueBASICS contains all of these ingredients in a simple daily pack.
TrueBOOST Metabolic support with L-Tyrosine	●	L-Tyrosine is essential for the formation of thyroid hormone. Low levels of this hormone are associated with an intolerance of cold temperatures, and frequently feeling cold, as well as weight gain, dry skin, hair loss, and/or constipation.
TrueB Formula High potency B complex	●	B vitamins are necessary for the production of thyroid hormone. Low levels of thyroid hormone are associated with feeling cold, slow metabolism, hair loss, and fatigue. B vitamins may assist with a reduction of these symptoms.
MEN'S HEALTH		
TrueBASICS	●	TrueBASICS contains ingredients necessary for a healthy immune system, high energy levels, and nutrient-deficiency prevention. TrueBASICS ensures the foundation of health. The grapeseed extract, vitamin E, zinc, selenium, B vitamins, fish oil, and vitamin A in this formula are all beneficial for the health of the prostate gland.
TruePROSTATE Nutritional support for prostate health	●	TruePROSTATE is designed to support prostate health. It contains a combination of vitamins, minerals, amino acids, nutrients, and herbs, such as saw palmetto, *Pygeum africanum,* and pumpkin seeds. Every man over 40 should take a prostate formula to ensure prostate health.
OPTIMAL WELLNESS		
TrueBASICS	●	TrueBASICS contains ingredients necessary for a healthy immune system, high energy levels, and nutrient-deficiency prevention. TrueBASICS ensures the foundation of health. Just one mineral or vitamin at lower than optimal levels can leave you at risk of fatigue or colds and flus — don't leave yourself lacking!

PRODUCT	RATING	WHY CHOOSE
TrueOMEGA Enteric-coated soft gels for cardiovascular health, brain health, and wellness	●	Fish oils can benefit almost every cell in the body. Supplements have been found to assist with weight loss, joint pain, heart health, brain health, mood, learning, memory, and digestive function. A minimum of 2 g should be taken daily for optimal results. Remember, your BASICS only contains 1 g.
TruePROTECT Basic antioxidant support	●	Taking antioxidant supplements is like putting money into the health bank for a rainy day. Antioxidants help to prevent cancer, aging, heart disease, Alzheimer's disease, and other illnesses associated with oxidative stress.
TrueCELL Coenzyme Q10 with lipoic acid	●	TruePROTECT and TrueCELL contain the most potent antioxidants available. If you are concerned with maintaining a healthy brain and heart (and preventing wrinkles too), you need to include this product in your daily supplement plan. TrueCELL can also prevent cellular damage due to excessive sugar intake, and the coenzyme Q10 improves energy by aiding cellular metabolism.
TrueLEAN III Weight loss, detox and cleaning fiber formula	●	A cleanse once or twice a year is a fantastic idea to reduce the toxic load of the body. It also prepares your body to accept the high quality supplements you will be adding as part of your Truestar Supplement Plan. Your liver and your digestive tract are key to good health and the maintenance of healthy body composition. Keep in mind that when you start a fat-loss program, your fat cells store a lot of waste products in the body. Taking this product will assist your system to cope with the cleanup!
PSYCHOLOGICAL HEALTH		
TrueBASICS	●	TrueBASICS contains ingredients necessary for a healthy immune system, high energy levels, and nutrient-deficiency prevention. TrueBASICS ensures the foundation of health. Taking vitamin C and vitamin E daily can reduce your risk of Alzheimer's disease by 58%! The fish oil and the grapeseed extract in this formula are protective to the brain cells and cognitive function, and the B vitamins assist with depression.

PRODUCT	RATING	WHY CHOOSE
TrueADAPT Ashwaganda stress support	●	Ashwaganda is unique in that it can be both stress supporting and energy-boosting. It is useful for anxiety because it increases the production of calming hormones.
TrueB Formula High-potency B complex	●	B vitamins can assist with depression, stress support, and improve energy levels.
TrueMOOD Standardized botanical extract of St. John's Wort in vegetarian capsules	●	TrueMOOD contains St. John's Wort, found to raise levels of serotonin, our 'feel-good' hormone, that is often deficient in cases of depression.
TrueOMEGA Enteric-coated soft gels for cardiovascular health, brain health, and wellness	●	DHA oils are highly concentrated within the brain, making them useful for the protection of brain structure and function.
TrueSUPPORT Botanical blend for healthy mental support and stress reduction with relora and vitamin B complex	●	TrueSUPPORT contains relora, found to lower cortisol levels, our long-term stress hormone, typically elevated in depression and anxiety.
SMOKING CESSATION		
TrueBASICS	●	Smoking increases your exposure to toxic compounds and your risk of cancer. You need more antioxidants. TrueBASICS contains selenium, zinc, vitamin A, vitamin E, grapeseed extract, and vitamin C, which may help to protect you from disease. However, quitting smoking is always your best source of health insurance.
TrueADAPT Ashwaganda stress support	●	Ashwaganda is unique in that it can be both stress-supporting and energy-boosting. It is useful for anxiety because it increases the production of calming hormones and may help to ease addictions and cravings.
TrueALLERFREE Quercetin-bromelain complex	●	TrueALLERFREE contains quercetin, vitamin C, and bromelain, which are excellent anti-inflammatory and antihistamine compounds for the health of the lungs and the immune system.

● Highly Recommended

● Beneficial

PRODUCT	RATING	WHY CHOOSE
TruePROTECT Basic antioxidant support	●	Smoking greatly increases your exposure to compounds that cause cancer, aging, and cellular damage. Taking TruePROTECT protects your cells, but your best defence is to quit smoking.
TrueSOOTHE Digestive healing and immunity support with DGL	●	DGL is healing and soothing to the mucus membranes of the mouth and is mildly cleansing for the lungs.
STRENGTH TRAINING		
TrueBASICS	●	Exercise elevates your nutrient needs as sweating increases the loss of many nutrients, such as the B vitamins and zinc, and the boost in metabolism increases your need for antioxidants. Vitamin E aids with recovery after exercises and calcium-magnesium is crucial for proper muscle growth, contraction, and relaxation. Do not leave your body lacking for vitamins, minerals, and antioxidants by missing your BASICS daily — your performance may suffer!
TrueBUILD Gastro-intestinal support with glutamine 500 mg capsules	●	L-Glutamine aids in the production of proteins, important for building muscle. It boosts growth hormone essential for muscle growth and repair and prevents the breakdown of muscle fibers.
TrueSTRENGTH Whey protein powder	●	Whey protein assists with lean muscle mass, aids recovery from exercise, maintains a healthy immune system, prevents the symptoms of over-training, and aids weight loss.
TrueSUPPORT Botanical blend for healthy mental support and stress reduction with relora and vitamin B complex	●	Relora, the herbal blend contained in TrueSUPPORT, helps to keep the body strong, healthy, and resilient during training. This product can be used to prevent increases in the stress hormone cortisol associated with over-training or with long, intense workouts. Cortisol suppresses the immune system and can damage muscle fibers, thereby inhibiting your ability to gain size.
TruePROTECT Basic antioxidant support	●	Exercise increases the need for extra antioxidant protection. Vitamins E and C, contained in this product, may also help to reduce soreness after exercise.

PRODUCT	RATING	WHY CHOOSE
STRESS		
TrueBASICS	●	TrueBASICS contains ingredients necessary for a healthy immune system, high energy levels, and nutrient-deficiency prevention. Taking this product daily ensures a strong foundation of health. It helps you stay healthy when stress, anxiety, overwork, or sleep deprivation begin to take their toll on your immune system. The fish oils contained in this formula protect the brain from the harmful effects of the stress hormone cortisol, while the calcium-magnesium ingredient is naturally calming and can improve your sleep.
TrueSUPPORT Botanical blend for healthy mental support and stress reduction with relora and vitamin B complex	●	TrueSUPPORT contains relora, found to lower cortisol levels, our long-term stress hormone. This herbal blend is calming without sedation and excellent for stress protection.
TrueB Formula High potency B complex	◉	Vitamin B supplements may assist with fatigue and energy levels.
TrueC	◉	Within 20 minutes of being under stress, vitamin C is depleted in the body. Vitamin C is necessary for a healthy immune system, collagen production, antioxidant protection and stress support.
WOMEN'S HEALTH		
TrueBASICS	●	TrueBASICS contains ingredients necessary for a healthy immune system, high energy levels, and nutrient-deficiency prevention. Taking this product daily is a great way to ensure the foundation of health. Also, the grapeseed extract, vitamin E, zinc, selenium, B vitamins, fish oil, and vitamin A in this formula are beneficial for breast health.
TrueMENO Comprehensive nutritional support during menopause	●	TrueMENO contains herbal ingredients that assist with the reduction of symptoms associated with changing levels of estrogen and progesterone in menopause. TrueMENO may offer a replacement to synthetic HRT, with the advice of your doctor.

PRODUCT	RATING	WHY CHOOSE
TrueB	●	B vitamins are important for the treatment and prevention of PMS and other women's health conditions associated with hormonal imbalance. Vitamin B-5 is especially important for stress support, while vitamin B-6 assists with hormone regulation, energy levels, stress support, and water retention.
TrueDESIRE for Women Libido boost formula	●	This product contains phytoestrogenic herbs to assist with the symptoms of a low libido, PMS, or hormonal imbalance.
TrueSUPPORT Botanical blend for healthy mental support and stress reduction with relora and vitamin B complex	●	TrueSUPPORT contains relora, an herbal blend that may assist with hot flashes, anxiety, sleep disruption, and abdominal weight gain associated with menopause. For sleep disruption, it is best to take 2 SUPPORT pills at bedtime and 1 in the morning.
WEIGHT LOSS PHASE I		
TrueBASICS	●	A deficiency of just one nutrient is enough to slow down your metabolism. Case in point: magnesium is involved in over 300 metabolic reactions in the body; B vitamins are crucial to the metabolism of carbohydrates, and fats and fish oils have been proven to assist a healthy body composition. TrueBASICS contains antioxidants (A, C, E, zinc, selenium and grapeseed extract). Antioxidant protection is essential in any weight-loss program because the fat cells release many stored toxins. The calcium in TrueBASICS, when taken regularly, has also been proven to cause weight loss.
TrueCRAVE	●	TrueCRAVE contains nutrients that assist with cravings during Phase I of our nutrition plan where carbohydrate intake is restricted. Carbohydrates are addictive, and we often crave them when we are under stress. CRAVE can also reduce stress-related eating patterns. Typically, cravings should subside after 2 weeks; however, you can continute to take this product longer.

PRODUCT	RATING	WHY CHOOSE
TrueLEAN III Weight loss, detox and cleaning fiber formula	●	Any effective weight-loss program should begin with detoxification of the liver and the digestive tract because these two organs are essential to healthy fat metabolism and waste removal. A detox also prepares your body for maximum benefits from the nutrients in your Truestar Supplement Plan. The fiber, herbs to simulate the thyroid gland (the master of our metabolic rate), diuretic herbs, and liver-cleansing formula in this pack can all assist with weight loss and can also prevent constipation, which commonly occurs in carbohydrate-restricted diets.
TrueABS Healthy insulin response and body composition support with conjugated linoleic acid and green tea	◐	TrueABS contains conjugated linoleic acid, a type of fatty acid supplement found to improve the body's response to insulin. In doing so, it has been proven to assist with fat loss and the maintenance of lean muscle mass. This product must be taken at a minimum dose of 4 pills per day for 3 months to be fully effective (optimal intake is 6 to 8 pills per day).
TrueLEAN II Weight management formula	◐	TrueLEAN assists with weight loss in a non-stimulating, safe, and effective manner by increasing metabolism, decreasing appetite, and improving the body's response to insulin. Because TrueLEAN II and III work on different mechanisms for weight loss, they both can be taken together to optimize your results.
TrueCARB Blocker	◐	When taken before meals that contain starch and fat, the herbs in CARB Blocker block the enzymes involved in the process of digestion of fats and carbohydrates. CARB Blocker contains ingredients to keep blood sugar levels low after meals, thereby assisting with the maintenance of low insulin levels. Because insulin is the hormonal signal that instructs the body to store energy as fat, keeping insulin levels low is helpful for weight loss.
TrueTHERMO	◐	TrueTHERMO is our thermogenic agent. Thermogenic products boost fat burning in the body and also improve metabolism in any phase of our weight-loss program. THERMO contains green tea and tyrosine, proven to assist with energy, stress, and fat loss during carbohydrate restriction. For maximum effect, this product is best taken before a workout.

PRODUCT	RATING	WHY CHOOSE
WEIGHT LOSS PHASE II		
TrueBASICS	●	A deficiency of just one nutrient is enough to slow down your metabolism. Case in point: magnesium is involved in over 300 metabolic reactions in the body; B vitamins are crucial to the metabolism of carbohydrates and fats; and fish oils have been proven to assist with healthy body composition. Do not leave yourself lacking! TrueBASICS contains antioxidants (Vitamin A, C, E, zinc, selenium, and grapeseed extract). Antioxidant protection is essential in any weight loss program because the fat cells release many stored toxins. The calcium in TrueBASICS, when taken regularly, has also been proven to cause weight loss.
TrueLEAN II Weight management formula	●	TrueLEAN III assists with weight loss in a non-stimulating, safe, and effective manner by increasing metabolism, decreasing appetite, and improving the body's response to insulin. This product should be taken along with CARB Blocker until your goal weight is achieved.
TrueCARB Blocker	●	When taken before meals that contain starch and fat, the herbs in CARB Blocker block the enzymes involved in the process of digestion of fats and carbohydrates. CARB Blocker contains ingredients to keep blood sugar levels low after meals, thereby assisting with the maintenance of low insulin levels. Because insulin is the hormonal signal that instructs the body to store energy as fat, keeping insulin levels low is helpful for weight loss. Along with TrueLEAN II, this product should be taken until your weight goal is achieved.
TrueABS Healthy insulin response and body composition support with conjugated linoleic acid and green tea	◉	TrueABS contains conjugated linoleic acid, a type of fatty acid supplement found to improve the body's response to insulin. In doing so, it has been proven to assist with fat loss and the maintenance of lean muscle mass. This product must be taken at a minimum dose of 4 four pills per day for 3 months to be fully effective (optimal intake is 6 to 8 pills per day).
TrueTHERMO	◉	TrueTHERMO is our thermogenic agent. Thermogenic products boost fat burning in the body and also improve metabolism in

PRODUCT	RATING	WHY CHOOSE
		any phase of our weight-loss program. THERMO contains green tea and tyrosine, proven to assist with energy, stress, and fat loss during carbohydrate restriction. For maximum effect, this product is best taken before a workout.
TrueLEAN III Weight loss, detox and cleaning fiber formula	◐	TrueLEAN III aids with weight loss and helps to prevent constipation, which commonly occurs in carbohydrate-restricted diets. The fiber assists with a feeling of fullness and improves digestive function. Two herbal ingredients simulate the thyroid gland (the master of our metabolic rate), diuretic herbs assist with weight gain related to water retention, and the liver-cleansing formula increases bile flow and assists with fat metabolism. For maximum weight-loss results, this product can be taken with TrueLEAN II because it works on different mechanisms in the body involved in weight loss.
SLEEP IMPROVEMENT		
TrueBASICS	●	TrueBASICS contains all of the vitamins and minerals necessary for good health along with fish oils that have a calming effect. The calcium-magnesium pills in this pack, when taken before bed, can help improve sleep, relax muscle tension, and calm the nervous system.
TrueSUPPORT Botanical blend for healthy mental support and stress reduction with relora and vitamin B complex	◐	TrueSUPPORT contains relora that assists with stress and disrupted sleep patterns. Individuals who are under stress may find that they have difficulty falling asleep, wake up too early, or tend to wake up between 2:00 a.m. and 4:00 a.m. Take 2 pills before bedtime and 1 in the morning on an empty stomach.
TrueCALM Calming herbal formula	◐	TrueCALM contains the calming herbs valerian, passion flower, hops, and skullcap, which improve sleeping patterns without side effects. This product is useful for individuals who have difficulty falling asleep or for people who complain about muscle tension or cramps. Take 3 pills before bedtime.
TrueZZZs — Melatonin	◐	Melatonin is a hormone necessary for healthy sleep patterns. This hormone naturally decreases as we age. This product is useful for sleeplessness in individuals over 45 years of age, and for treating jet lag.

PRODUCT	RATING	WHY CHOOSE
THE TRUESTAR CLEANSE AND DETOX		
TrueBASICS	◐	A deficiency of just one nutrient is enough to slow down your metabolism. Case in point: magnesium is involved in over 300 metabolic reactions in the body; B vitamins are crucial to the metabolism of carbohydrates and fats; and fish oils have been proven to assist with healthy body composition. Do not leave yourself lacking! TrueBASICS contains antioxidants (vitamins A, C, E, zinc, selenium, and grapeseed extract). Antioxidant protection is essential in any weight loss program because the fat cells release many stored toxins. The calcium in TrueBASICS, when taken regularly, has also been proven to cause weight loss.
TrueLEAN III	●	TrueLEAN III contains a liver-cleansing formula with herbs that improves the flow of bile, aids liver cell regeneration, and reduces elevated liver enzymes. Improving the flow of bile is necessary for bowel function, waste removal, and hormonal balance. The fiber in this formula also assists with bowel cleansing.
TrueDOPHILUS Beneficial flora for healthy intestinal function	●	During any cleanse, it is essential to have healthy bacterial balance in the gut for regular bowel movements and to improve immunity and hormonal balance. It is crucial to avoid becoming constipated during a cleanse (think about all the toxins your liver and body have prepared for removal that can become stagnant in the colon and potentially become re-absorbed). Constipation contributes to headaches, fatigue, chemical sensitivities, and PMS. Acidophilus, the good bacteria in the bowel, can greatly assist in waste removal.
TrueC	◐	Taking vitamin C during a cleanse can assist your body with the process of detoxification and can help prevent detox symptoms, such as headaches, fatigue, irritability, or constipation.
TrueB	◐	TrueB can assist energy levels during a detox and aid with the process of carbohydrate metabolism. Try taking it at lunch time with a vitamin C tablet when you are doing your cleanse. It helps to keep you going throughout the day.

PRODUCT	RATING	WHY CHOOSE
TrueOMEGA Enteric-coated soft gels for cardiovascular health, brain health, and wellness	◐	TrueOMEGA should be part of any wellness or detoxification plan because the fish oils contained in this product can benefit almost all the cells in the body. Fish oils are naturally anti-inflammatory agents and can decrease joint pain and stiffness, aid bowel function, improve mood, and aid with fat loss.
HEALTHY LIVER PLAN		
TrueLEAN III	◐	TrueLEAN III contains an herbal liver-cleansing formula to improve the flow of bile and aid liver cell regeneration. It may also help reduce elevated liver enzymes.
TrueBASICS	◐	A deficiency of just one vitamin or mineral can interfere with proper liver and metabolic function. BASICS contains all the supplements you need to ensure your needs are met daily.
TrueC	●	Vitamin C has been shown to protect the cells of the liver and to aid in detoxification.
FIBROMYALGIA		
TrueBASICS	●	The calcium-magnesium in TrueBASICS can reduce muscle pain and establish normal sleeping patterns. Low levels of magnesium are common in fibromyalgia — possibly a causal factor of fatigue and muscle pain. Exercise is indicated for fibromyalgia sufferers, but care must be used to avoid over-training. The vitamin E in BASICS helps to prevent excess soreness after exercise. The potent multivitamin will prevent nutrient deficiency caused by chronic pain and stress of illness. The fish oils in BASICS are natural anti-inflammatory compounds, valuable for reducing pain and stiffness. The fish oils also assist with depression or anxiety commonly associated with chronic pain.
TrueB	◐	Fatigue is common in fibromyalgia. B vitamins can help to stabilize energy levels.
TrueCRAVE	◐	TrueCRAVE contains 5HTP, a precursor to serotonin. Low levels of 5HTP are associated with the muscle pain and headaches of fibromyalgia. The glutamine and other minerals in this product may also assist with muscle soreness.

PRODUCT	RATING	WHY CHOOSE
TrueOMEGA Enteric-coated soft gels for cardiovascular health, brain health, and wellness	●	TrueOMEGA should be part of any wellness plan because the fish oils contained in this product can benefit almost all the cells in the body. Fish oils are naturally anti-inflammatory agents and can improve joint pain and stiffness, aid bowel function, improve mood, and assist with fat loss. Fish oils are beneficial for treating depression, anxiety, pain, sleep disruption, and digestive upset, often associated with fibromyalgia.
TrueMSM Collagen and joint support with Methylsulfonylmethane	●	MSM is a natural anti-inflammatory compound that may ease the pain of fibromyalgia. The sulfur in this product can assist with healthy liver function and detoxification. Cleansing and detox are also useful in treating many cases of fibromyalgia.
TrueLEAN III	●	TrueLEAN III assists with detoxification of the body. Cleansing and detox also assist with many cases of fibromyalgia.
TrueTHERMO	●	Many people with fibromyalgia have chronic fatigue. THERMO provides a quick energy boost, especially before a workout.
TrueSUPPORT Botanical blend for healthy mental support and stress reduction with relora and vitamin B complex	●	TrueSUPPORT assists with elevated levels of stress hormone that may occur with chronic pain. It may also help with the sleep disruption, depression, and/or anxiety often associated with fibromyalgia.

POLYCYSTIC OVARIAN DISEASE (PCOS)

PRODUCT	RATING	WHY CHOOSE
TrueBASICS	●	The calcium-magnesium combination in the BASICS can assist with healthy hormonal balance, menstrual cramping, reducing the signs of PMS, and weight loss. The vitamin E and grapeseed extract components are good antioxidants to help reduce cancer risks. The fish oil contained in TrueBASICS assists with weight loss, inflammation, and hormonal imbalance.
TrueABS Conjugated linoleic acid	●	TrueABS works by improving the body's response to insulin. PCOS, associated with insulin resistance, can be improved with supplements of CLA when taken regularly. Lowering levels of insulin can also protect against breast cancer. The risk of breast cancer is higher in PCOS patients if their care is not properly managed.

PRODUCT	RATING	WHY CHOOSE
TrueB	●	B vitamins assist with hormonal balance, depression, anxiety, and metabolism. They are also beneficial for women on the birth control pill because the pill depletes folic acid and other nutrients in the body. Many women with PCOS resort to taking the pill to establish a regular menstrual cycle, but there are natural alternatives.
TrueDOPHILUS Beneficial flora for healthy intestinal function	●	Many women who have PCOS take the birth control pill, which alters healthy bacterial balance in the digestive tract. The good bacteria contained in TrueDOPHILUS is important for hormonal balance because it is involved in the metabolism of estrogen in the body. DOPHILUS also assists in regular bowel movements, central to wellness and health.
TrueLEAN II	●	TrueLEAN II contains ingredients to assist with weight loss and healthy blood sugar balance by improving the body's response to insulin, thereby lowering insulin levels, the hormone that tells the body to store energy as fat and is a dieter's nemesis. Weight loss is crucial for all PCOS patients because a reduction in body weight by a mere 13% helps to increase fertility and menstrual regularity significantly.
TrueLEAN III	●	Healthy hormonal balance is directly linked to liver function and bowel health. This product can help with liver and digestive tract cleansing. It also helps to reduce acne breakouts, common in PCOS.
TruePROSTATE Nutritional support for prostate health with saw palmetto	●	Many women with PCOS have abnormally high testosterone levels. Taking saw palmetto daily can help to reduce elevated testosterone levels and to decrease many of the symptoms associated with high testosterone levels, such as acne, hair loss, weight gain and abnormal hair growth.
TrueCARB Blocker	●	CARB Blocker keeps insulin and blood sugar levels low after a meal. This decreases the hormonal imbalances and weight gain associated with PCOS. It helps with weight loss — a key component for fertility and for PCOS patients.

Tips for Taking Vitamins

Starting a supplement program can be challenging. Once you have tackled the huge task of determining which products to buy, you then have to figure out what dose to take, when to take them, and what combinations work best! You can have the best program in the world, but unless you develop a system to get in the habit of taking vitamins, your money will be wasted. Taking vitamins is like most new things in life — once you do it 21 times, it becomes a habit. Before you know it, you will notice the difference between how you feel throughout the day when you take your vitamins and when you don't. Your belief in the importance of vitamins for your optimal wellness will help to keep you on track. Go back and read the section on why we should take vitamins if you feel your motivation is lagging.

> Taking vitamins is like most new things in life — once you do it 21 times, it becomes a habit.

How to Remember to Take Your Vitamins

- **Out of sight — out of mind!** Keep them on the counter, in the bathroom, at the office (5 times per week is better than none!).
- **K.I.S.S.** Write on the top with a marker, "# per day." Or write down your supplement schedule by time of day. You can also use the sample daily vitamin schedule provided here to assist you.
- **Keep organized:** Group products (with food, without food, before bed, on rising, once a day, twice a day) to keep yourself organized.
- **Put a reminder in your calendar for each day of the week:** This is especially helpful if different vitamins are taken on different days.

When to Take Your Supplements

VITAMINS AND MINERALS: Generally, most vitamins are best tolerated and absorbed when taken with food. The enzymes and hydrochloric acid released with the intake of food will aid absorption and also prevent nausea, sometimes experienced if certain vitamins and supplements are taken on an empty stomach.

Vitamins and minerals are best taken in dosages spaced throughout the day across several meals rather than all at once to maintain proper levels of

	Supplement	Sun	Mon	Tues	Wed	Thurs	Fri	Sat
Your Truestar Supplement Program Schedule								
Before breakfast (empty stomach)	TrueLEAN	✓	✓					
With breakfast	TrueBASICS	✓	✓					
Before lunch (empty stomach)	TrueLEAN	✓						
With lunch	TrueCARDIO	✓						
Before dinner (empty stomach)								
With dinner	TrueOMEGA	✓						
Before bedtime (empty stomach)	TrueCALM	✓						

Log on to www.truestarhealth.com to create a personal vitamin plan based on your weight-loss goals, physical activity level, and current health status.

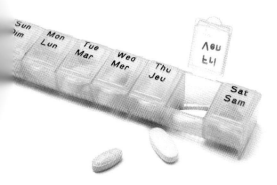

CALCIUM EXCEPTION: Studies suggest that calcium is best taken before bed to have the most beneficial effect on building bone strength and mass. Taking a calcium-magnesium supplement at bedtime may also help with your sleep because it is a natural muscle relaxant and can calm the mind. Aim to take one dose with a meal and the other before bed.

ZINC CAUTION: Taking too much zinc at once can cause stomach cramping and nausea. Some people can tolerate the RDA (15 mg) at one time and no more. Zinc is beneficial for a number of conditions and the unpleasant effects can be lessened by taking it with food. More than 100 mg of zinc should not be taken in one day; otherwise, immune system function may be suppressed.

Most vitamins are best tolerated and absorbed when taken with food.

intake. If you must take them all at once, do so your with largest meal. Read labels and if ingredients in products overlap, take them at separate times during the day. For example, it is much better to take your B complex separate from your multivitamin, which will also contain B vitamins. This will keep your levels steady.

FAT SOLUBLE VITAMINS: Note that vitamins A, D, E, and K are fat soluble vitamins that require fat, either animal or vegetable, to be present in the stomach for them to be optimally absorbed. Coenzyme Q10 also requires fat to be properly absorbed. These products must be taken with meals.

WATER SOLUBLE VITAMINS: Water soluble vitamins, such as the B vitamins and vitamin C, do not require fat to be optimally absorbed by the body. However, B vitamins require an acidic environment to be absorbed, so are best taken with meals. If you are currently taking antacids, H2 blockers, or other drugs that deplete stomach acid, you may have a decreased ability to absorb B vitamins.

HERBAL REMEDIES: Unless specifically noted on the label or instructed to do so by your doctor, herbal remedies are generally best taken away from food for maximum absorption and effect. This means 20 to 30 minutes before meals or 1½ to 2 hours after.

ESSENTIAL FATTY ACIDS: Most people prefer to take these with meals, although it is not necessary. You can keep your essential fatty acids in the refrigerator or freezer to maintain their freshness, especially if they are in liquid form. Oils in liquid form usually only keep for about 4 to 6 weeks after opening. Capsules may not need to be refrigerated, but be sure to keep them away from heat and sunlight.

If the bottle smells fishy, don't take them — it means they are no longer fresh! Try to take a capsule of vitamin E at the same time as your fats to prevent oxidization. If taking ground flaxseed, purchase a product that is vacuum packed and keep it in the freezer after opening. Even better — grind your own. The seeds have advantages over the pure flax oil because they contain fiber and ligands, which are cancer protecting and hormone balancing.

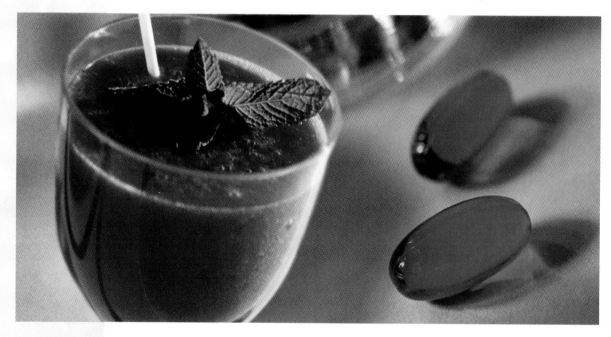

Tricks for Taking Vitamins

Some people have success swallowing pills better in a thicker liquid, such as yogurt or a smoothie, than in water.

Most people have few problems, if any, when taking vitamins, but sometimes minor complaints may arise.

DIFFICULTY SWALLOWING: For those who find it difficult to swallow pills, consider opening up capsules, crushing tablets, or blending them into a smoothie to drink. This does not reduce their effectiveness. Many supplements may be available in user-friendly powder or liquid form.

Using an old-fashioned mortar and pestle, crush the tablets and combine the powder with oatmeal, yogurt, smoothies, or diluted juice. Some people have success swallowing pills easier in a thicker liquid, such as yogurt or a smoothie, than in water.

NAUSEA: This can be fairly common if vitamins are taken on an empty stomach. Taking your supplements with food should do the trick. The nausea is often a result of zinc, B complex, or 5-HTP.

LOOSE STOOLS: Loose stools can be caused by various supplements. It is best to reduce the dose or to stop the product until the digestive symptoms settle down. Then build the dosage up to bowel tolerance or re-introduce the products one at a time.

YELLOW URINE: This is a normal reaction to taking B vitamins. Yellow urine is nothing to be concerned about if you are drinking enough water daily, although we still get tons of questions about this all the time!

NIACIN FLUSH: This can occur when taking B vitamins or, in very sensitive individuals, when taking a multivitamin containing niacin (vitamin B-3). The flush is characterized by itching, dilation of the blood vessels causing reddening, tingling in the skin, and possibly a headache because of the increased blood flow to the head. This is harmless — but can be very disconcerting. Drink water and take your B vitamins with food. The flush is dose dependent, so sometimes breaking the B complex in half and taking it at separate times rather than all at once can eliminate the problem. Note: if you experience wheezing, it is likely due to an allergy and you should see your doctor.

BURPING FISH OILS: Some people experience a reflux or repeating taste of fish oils. Swallow your oils right at the beginning of your largest meal. If it continues, keep

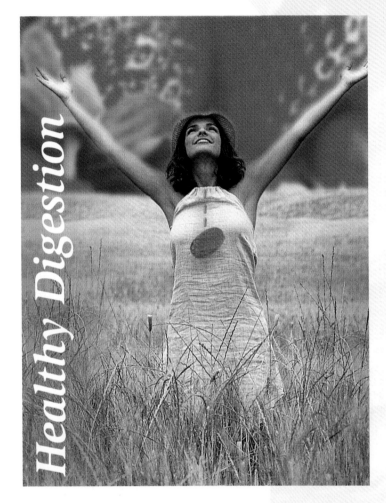

Healthy Digestion

the bottle of fish oils in the freezer and continue to take the fish oils with food. Somehow, freezing the fish oil seems to reduce the problem.

ELIMINATION: A good general rule to follow if you encounter any of these problems is to stop everything for a day or two. When the symptom clears up, add the products back one at a time to determine which product, if at all, may be causing the reaction.

Yellow urine is nothing to be concerned about if you are drinking enough water.

"Life has to be lived. That's all there is to it. "
Eleanor Roosevelt

Safety Concerns

Supplements are remarkably safe. One study of acute or chronic overdoses, with more than 40,000 exposures, reported only one death and eight major adverse outcomes.

However, it is true that some vitamins and minerals can be toxic when taken in excess. Iron-containing vitamins are the most toxic, especially in pediatric acute ingestions, as well as in men. Fat-soluble vitamins (vitamin A, D, E, and K) are more dangerous as they can be stored in the body and accumulate.

Vitamins can also react adversely with some medications, causing health prob-

lems, while some are contraindicated for use with other health products or for specific health conditions.

So, you do need to exercise caution when taking supplements, especially if you are using medications, are pregnant or breastfeeding, or have a serious medical condition. You should always check with your doctor or pharmacist before taking any nutritional supplement.

Toxicity

Toxicity is a condition where the concentration in the body of any one mineral or vitamin is abnormally high, resulting in an adverse effect on health. An overdose (excessive amount) of a nutrient can result in toxicity either acutely or chronically (over a period of time). Look for general signs and symptoms of toxicity of vitamins and let your doctor know if you suspect a problem.

- Nonspecific symptoms, such as nausea, vomiting, diarrhea, and rash, are common with any acute or chronic vitamin overdose.
- Vitamin-caused symptoms may be secondary to those associated with additives (mannitol, for example), colorings, or binders. These symptoms usually are not severe.

In some circles, the myth persists that vitamins are not good for your health and can cause death if overdosed.

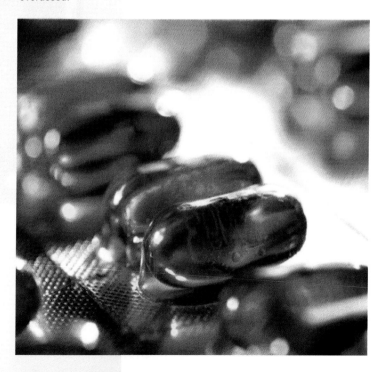

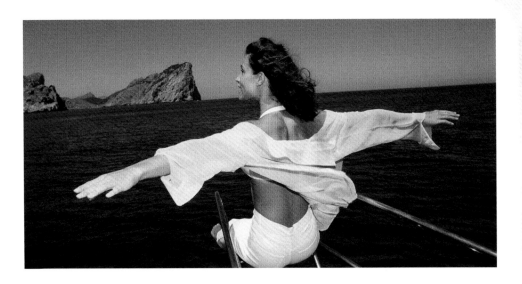

Adverse Interactions

Taking a vitamin or supplement with a drug could have a negative result. It may occur because the vitamin enhances the activity of the drug (which may result in toxicity) or because the supplement interferes with the absorption or action of the drug (lessening its action in the body).

Contraindications

Sometimes a vitamin or supplement should not be taken with another drug, herb, or natural health product because there is a potential for a negative result.

For more information on vitamin toxicity, interactions, and contraindications, log on at www.truestarhealth.com.

If you exercise, live in a city, drink caffeine, consume alcohol, take medications, or are under stress, your need for nutritional supplements is much higher.

The Truestar Way …

We believe nutritional supplements are one of the five keys to total health and weight loss the Truestar way. Taking supplements daily may result in increased vitality, energy, immunity, and wellness. If you exercise, live in a city, drink caffeine, consume alcohol, take medications, or are under stress, your need for nutritional supplements is much higher. A deficiency of just one nutrient is enough to cause fatigue and frequent infections, resulting in a poor sense of well-being and even an increase in your risk of heart disease or cancer. Taking supplements is all about preserving health before treating disease.

Regardless of age, each of us can benefit from the addition of vitamins to our daily lifestyle.

Attitude

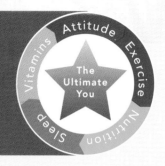

Give Me Good Attitude Anytime!

Tim Mulcahy, CEO

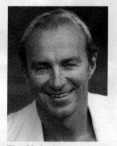

Tim Mulcahy

I had not made learning about attitude a formal component of my life until near disaster struck a decade ago.

In the direct sales business, having a good attitude every day is vital. 'Not giving up when the going gets tough' was an attitude I developed as a young man when I sold door to door. While I read a few motivational books, like *Think and Grow Rich* by Napoleon Hill, and listened to Anthony Robbins' motivational CDs, I had not made learning about attitude a formal component of my life until near disaster struck a decade ago.

At the time, I owned a company with my brother that marketed telephone services for STN Long Distance. We were doing really well. We sold about 300,000 contracts for STN over a year and were owed close to $4.5 million in residual payments. However, STN had grown too quickly and ended up filing for bankruptcy, leaving us without work — and without much money. We tried to sue but didn't have an "in case of bankruptcy" clause in our contract.

Initially depressed by this loss, I tried to rebound by going back into the water filter business, but couldn't get excited about it. I put up my antennae for new ventures. Because there had been a lot of news about home invasions and break-ins, I thought the timing would be right for the home-alarm business. My brother and I tried to start our own alarm company, but soon realized we were under-capitalized, so I approached a wealthy acquaintance with our business plan. With his capital and a verbal agreement to split the profits 50/50, we set off to build another new business. But when it came time to sign the partnership agreement, our 'partner' asked for 62.5%. We didn't have a lot of choice in the matter and signed.

These financial setbacks took a toll on me, affecting not only my business life but also my personal life. Each day at the office, bickering with our partner ate up my time and energy, leaving little for after business hours. I knew I had to make a change. I remember picking up *The 7 Habits of Highly Effective People*, the now

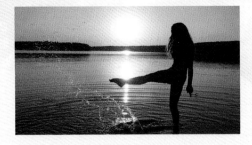

legendary book by Stephen Covey. Reading the preface and first chapter on "being proactive" shifted my attitude. I soon started looking for ways to improve myself personally and professionally.

Stephen Covey tells the story of Victor Frankl, who witnessed the execution of his parents, wife, and children in the Nazi concentration camps. Despite this nightmare, Frankl chose to be proactive and became somewhat of a motivational guru to the other prisoners. Even the guards would listen to him. In the end, he somehow managed to escape and wrote his classic book, *Man's Search for Meaning*. As a psychiatrist, Frankl pioneered an approach called logotherapy or responsibility therapy for responding positively to all events in your life.

When I read his story, I really felt like my response to my troubles was as foolish as a baby crying over spilled milk. This was truly a profound moment in my life. I decided then and there that I was going to shine from the inside out. Whether or not the sun was shining in my life or not, I was going to make it shine. We turned Neighborhood Protection Services into a very successful company, and since that day in August 1995, I have committed myself to listening to motivational audios and reading life-improvement books. As motivational guru Zig Ziglar says, "Motivation is like bathing; you need it daily."

Attitude is finally starting to gain a lot of respect when it comes to personal health.

Many healthcare professionals agree that physical disease or being "dis-at-ease" can manifest in your mind, too. This mind-body connection has become the subject of several best-selling books by well-known authors, such as Deepak Chopra and Carolyn Myss. They have helped me to understand that when, for example, I do catch a cold, it invariably happens during a time when my mental and emotional systems are weak or compromised.

I feel that keeping a positive attitude, more than anything in our daily life, is the key to maximizing our potential. Attitude became the next principle of the Truestar way to total health.

As motivational guru Zig Ziglar says, "Motivation is like bathing; you need it daily."

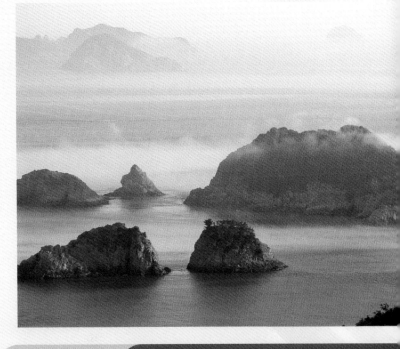

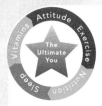

Attitude... the Truestar Way

Tim Mulcahy

Teaching Attitude

I'm always surprised that attitude is not something taught in our educational systems. The trigonometry and physics that I was taught and my children are learning may be of marginal value for the majority of adults, but attitude building techniques, such as goal-setting and positive self-talk, along with being grateful and remaining non-judgmental, would be extremely beneficial if introduced to young minds and young bodies at an early age. They are such great habits to develop.

The following Truestar attitude program can be adopted by all age groups and will have an immediate positive impact on your life. If one of your personal goals is to lose weight, a good attitude can play an important role. Zig Ziglar says that people lose more weight listening to his CDs than any weight loss program. I believe him. You can lose weight by taking

responsibility for doing so and using goal-setting techniques, along with positive self-talk. If you are motivated, you are generating a lot of mental energy from both your mind and soul. This mind-body-spirit synergy will affect your metabolism in a positive way, creating a higher metabolism. (My wife says that sometimes when I'm lying awake in bed, she can feel the bed vibrating from my thinking.) A depressed person is likely to have a slower metabolism.

The Truestar Life Improvement Program is the first and only on-line daily success habit coach. Log on at www.truestarhealth.com. We will teach you the necessary skills to create a life full of the happiness and success you desire.

Our program will help you discover your passion and purpose for life in our complex universe.

> When I do catch a cold, it invariably happens during a time when my mental and emotional systems are weak or compromised.

> "Everything can be taken from a man but . . . the last of the human freedoms — to choose one's attitude in any given set of circumstances; to choose one's own way."   Victor Frankl

The Truestar Life Improvement Program

At Truestar, we have developed 12 habits to improve your attitude and ensure daily success in achieving your goals, including everyone's goal of good health and lifelong wellness. We sometimes call this program the 12 habits of highly healthy people, paying respect to Stephen Covey's ground-breaking and highly influential book, *The 7 Habits of Highly Effective People.*

1. Gratitude

Gratitude is one of the easiest ways to improve your attitude; it doesn't take a lot of time and it doesn't cost any money. Our time on the planet is limited. Most of us are continually bogged down with projects, relationships, financial worries, and so on. In reality, the only people without problems are 6 feet under. How you deal with problems in your own life will determine your day-to-day level of happiness. Being grateful each and every day is a simple, immediate method to generate happiness.

As we begin to acknowledge the opportunities and blessings in each experience, we discover a profound, simple key: the power of lovingly accepting everything and everyone as is. Affix your days with a loving acceptance of life, dismiss fear-based attitudes, and discover how liberating it is to live without judgment, in complete appreciation of the perfection of everything and everyone.

When you are thankful for everything in your life, you will want to enrich the lives of others so they may be as thankful as you are. In this way,

your gratitude promotes an attitude of giving. Whether your gifts are material or verbal, or even if you give a thought, you will be touched as you bring smiles to the faces of others.

Gratitude Rituals

The following gratitude rituals will have an immediate impact on your life. Although the Truestar Way directs you to do this first thing in the morning and before bed, if you find yourself extremely stressed anytime during the day, this ritual will be helpful.

Morning Ritual

When you awaken, take 5 minutes to count your blessings, including your health, the special people in your life, and even the fact that you have been granted another day to make a difference. Along with your morning gratitude, make a commitment to greet each day and the people you encounter with love in your heart. As we rush through each day and get caught up in daily demands, we forget to stop and recognize the wonderful opportunities we have, the true miracle of simply being on the planet and having the opportunity to make a difference just by greeting the people we meet with love in our hearts. By acknowledging the amazing natural universe that surrounds us, we start each day with a more positive outlook. Just spending 5 minutes each morning being grateful, rather than lamenting, "Not another day

at work," can dramatically improve your attitude for the day.

Evening Gratitude

Being grateful for simply being granted another day is a humble yet powerful skill of personal development. A 5-minute bedtime review of the people, opportunities, and even challenges you have been blessed with allows you to put the day into a positive perspective, leading to a calm state and preparing you for a quality night's sleep.

Attitude Aids for Gratitude
- *The Seven Spiritual Laws of Success* by Deepak Chopra
- *The Greatest Salesman in the World* by Og Mandino
- *Get the Edge* by Anthony Robbins

> Just spending 5 minutes each morning being grateful, rather than lamenting, "Not another day at work," can dramatically improve your attitude for the day.

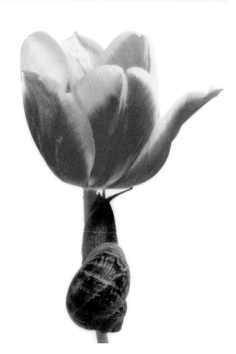

2. Responsibility

Responsibility is your ability to respond directly and honestly to any given circumstance. Often responsibility is mistaken for blame, guilt, or shame, when actually accepting responsibility shows discipline and maturity. Accepting responsibility allows you to be in control of every situation. You know that the outcome of the situation is based on your response to it.

Responsibility is an attitude that is not very well understood, however. Visionaries, such as Stephen Covey and Victor Frankl, counsel that only when you truly take responsibility for all your actions, can you start to gain control of your life. When I was recently listening to a Brian Tracy audio in my car, I first heard someone say that responsibility was more important than goal-setting for being successful. "If you don't take responsibility for everything that happens to you when taking action to achieve your goals," Brian Tracy says, "how can you be certain of achieving them?"

Responsible for Ourselves and for Others

"God helps those who help themselves," the bible says. For religious or spiritual persons who believe in a higher power (as do I), this statement is all about responsibility. If you truly want to help others, you have to take responsibility for your actions and help yourself first. A leading cancer clinic found that cancer patients who take responsibility for their disease have a far greater response to treatment than those who do not accept responsibility.

Taking responsibility for your actions, reactions, and results in life is the key for opening the door to life improvement.

Responsibility Self-Talk

This daily self-talk statement will help to condition attitude by developing the important skill of accepting responsibility for your actions, reactions, and results.

I accept total responsibility for my actions, reactions, and outcomes today and every day for the rest of my life. I understand that by accepting responsibility for my success and failures on a day-to-day basis, I take control of my life and am able to accept merit in regard to my success. Also, by accepting responsibility for my failures, I am able to learn and change as I realize that failure is an event, not a person. By accepting responsibility, I can change my actions, reactions, and outcomes in the future. I also realize that failure to accept responsibility leaves me powerless and without control to take life into my own hands.

> Taking responsibility for your actions, reactions, and results in life is the key for opening the door to life improvement.

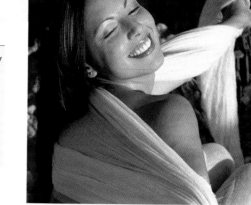

3. Laughing

Our actions can control our emotions; if you are feeling down, find a way to laugh and watch your emotions quickly change for the better!

Laugh and the world laughs with you! Although it is important to be serious and focused on many key areas of your life, having a good laugh and enjoying the journey to success, not just the destination, is proven to be extremely good for your health. One scientific study shows that three 5-second laughs each day may ward off illness by strengthening the body's immune system. Having a good sense of humor and not taking yourself too seriously are also leadership traits and a catalyst for quality relationships.

Lack of laughter can breed depression, which is merely anger without enthusiasm. Our actions can control our emotions; if you are feeling down, find a way to laugh and watch your emotions quickly change for the better! Watch a funny television show or movie; read comics or a joke book; associate with people with a sense of humor that you enjoy.

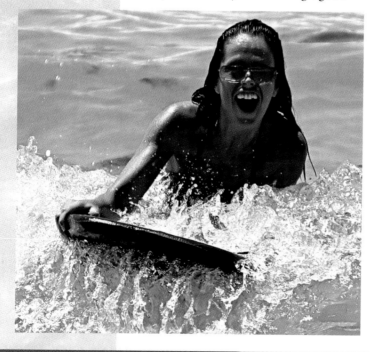

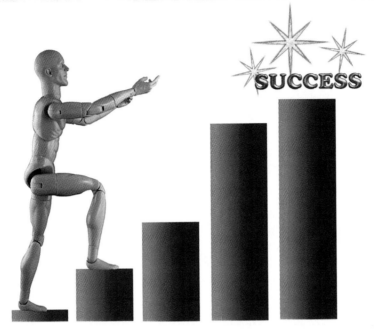

4. Goal Setting

Setting goals is a truly magical habit, a must for success in any area of your life. Living life without clear goals is like driving your car without a road map. Imagine being invited to someone's country home for the weekend without being given a map or directions. How long would it take you to find the home? You'd end up driving aimlessly around the countryside all weekend and never arrive at your destination. As silly as that sounds, people who live their lives without a formal goals program are no less silly.

Many years ago, the value of goal setting was studied at Yale University using the graduating class of 1953. The 400 graduating students were asked to write out a life-long plan that they intended to follow. Out of the 400, only 12 students or 3% of the total actually submitted a plan. Apparently, the others did not, either because they hadn't set any life-long goals or didn't want to take the time to do so. When the class had a reunion 20 years later and the '53 class was surveyed to see if they were happy with their lives, the 3% who had set goals seemed happier than the 97% who had not. While this observation about levels of happiness was somewhat unsophisticated and subjective, what could be objectively substantiated is that the 3% who had set long-term goals had a higher net worth than the other 97% combined!

Setting goals is a
truly magical
habit, a must for
success in any
area of your life.

Log on to www.truestarhealth.com to create a personal goal setting plan based on your weight-loss goals, physical activity level, and current heath status.

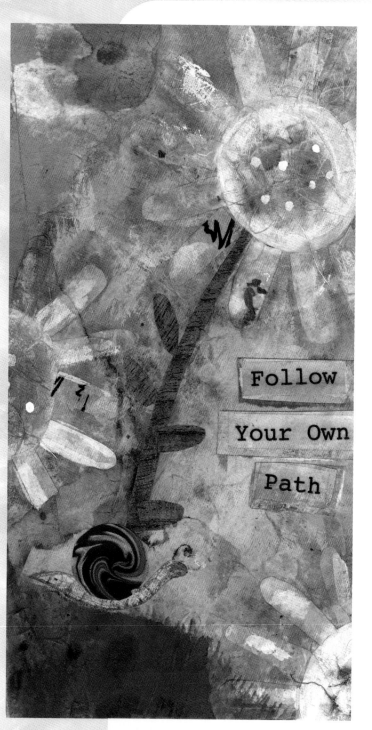

Follow

Your Own

Path

Hurricane Attitude

Goal setting is a ritual activity in my life. I always combine goal setting with visualization to maximize the intensity so I can focus on my outcomes. Back in August 1995 when I resolved to produce my own "sunshine," I wrote down 10 goals I wanted to achieve, including a financial goal I had no idea how to reach. By Christmas, I had reached 9 out of 10 goals, including the financial goal. The remaining goal was achieved a few years later, when I not only had the satisfaction of reaching my goal but also the thrill of motivating others to achieve theirs.

That magical experience in goal setting for me came when I was helping to coach an AAA PeeWee boys hockey team. AAA is the highest level. My friend Pete Bobechko had been a successful minor hockey coach for some time, and when he asked me to help him coach his team, I said "yes" immediately. Coaching minor hockey at that level was the one goal that I had yet to achieve from my list of 10.

The name of the team was the Halton Hurricanes. The team had never won a league championship or made it past the first round of the playoffs. The Hurricanes had placed last and second last in the two previous seasons. We had our work cut out for us.

When we chose the kids during try-outs that would make the team, several parents weren't too happy with some of the choices. We cut 8 boys who had played on the team the previous year and brought up 8 AA players, considered by

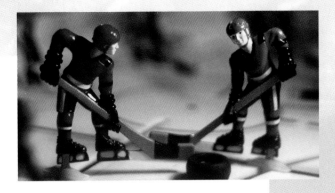

many of the parents to be inferior. One of the parents told Pete and me that he didn't think we would win one game all year. That was no deterrent to Pete, who at the first team meeting and throughout the season kept telling the boys to make sure they had a place cleared off on their shelf to showcase a championship trophy.

Pete is a great motivator. I taught motivation for a living. Our other coach and our friend, Timmy Harnett, is also an energetic man, so we didn't lack inspiration. The season started off slowly, as we only managed to post 3 wins, 6 losses, and 3 ties after the first 12 games, though some of the losses were very close. I decided it was time to implement a goal-setting program I had been working on for these 12-year-old boys.

I made up some goal-setting sheets for the boys to fill out and asked them to tape them to their wall in their bedroom. Each boy had to bring me a photograph of the goal-setting sheet taped to his wall, where he could review it daily. On this sheet, they had to state five team goals and five personal achievement goals for the season. Prior to each game, they had to fill out a sheet with five team goals and five personal goals for that game.

After the goal-setting sessions began, the team posted a record of 13 wins, 1 loss, and 7 ties. In the last game of the season, we beat our nemesis, Grey Bruce (a team that we had not beaten in the previous 2 years in over 10 meetings), 8-1. We ended up finishing 3rd in the league, but won in the playoffs to become the league champions, the first time ever for this team.

We also won a major tournament in Peterborough that year, something the team had never achieved, and the following year, we were invited to the Quebec PeeWee tournament, considered the closest thing to a PeeWee world championship. We made it to the finals but lost to the Czech Republic, a stunning showing for a team that "wouldn't win a game." We also won the league championship the following year. Not bad for a team that was not considered to be a contender.

That was one of the most magical changes I've seen deriving from the power of goal setting. More than once, my fellow coaches and I concluded that goal setting and many other attitude enhancing tools should be taught formally in schools beginning at a young age so that our kids could learn how to take positive control of their lives. The word "curriculum" means "running of life." What better curriculum is there than teaching life-preparing power skills like goal setting? One of my new personal goals is to see that happen!

> What better curriculum is there than teaching life-preparing power skills like goal setting?

Rules of Goal Setting

There are useful rules for goal setting. Let's consider them and where you can find the best tools to get those goals identified, articulated, and put into action. A goals program can make major problems easier to deal with, and minor problems can be handled routinely because you have the bigger picture in mind.

☐ Set realistic goals that you can achieve.

☐ Once you reach your goal, set a new one at a higher level.

☐ Review your goals throughout the day.

To develop a personalized goal-setting program, see www.truestarhealth.com. We offer the best interactive program for setting goals that is available online.

ATTITUDE AIDS FOR GOAL SETTING

☐ Anthony Robbins' *Personal Power* is the best goal-setting audio series that I've listened to and can be of great help. Robbins' personal story on how goal setting changed his life is very powerful.

☐ Zig Ziglar's audio *Goals Program* can't but help you achieve your goals. It's also a great easy-listening motivational program.

5. Daily Motivational Input

Daily motivational input is also key to building happiness in life. As Zig Ziglar says about motivation, "You need it daily or you'll get stinkin' thinkin.'"

Attending seminars given by motivational speakers, like Zig Ziglar, can be uplifting, but for some people it can also be overkill. Too much information loaded in too quickly can lessen the effect. Gradual input and absorption may be more effective.

Try reading a motivational book of your choice for 15 to 30 minutes in the morning. It's an excellent way to enhance your day. If, like many of us, your morning schedule is busy, we suggest listening to an audio tape or CD while traveling. Through audio

university, an average commuter can learn to the level of a basic university degree in 4 to 5 years of urban commuting.

Even if you only experience 30 minutes of motivational learning a day, your attitude will improve dramatically, helping you realize your true potential. For quicker conditioning and improvement, we suggest 30 minutes of motivational input in the morning and 30 minutes later in the day.

Listening to or reading motivational materials has created dramatic improvements in my life, financially, mentally, and spiritually. I currently listen to motivational audios at least an hour a day. I highly recommend Zig Ziglar's audio,

Even if you only experience 30 minutes of motivational learning a day, your attitude will improve dramatically, helping you realize your true potential.

Strategies for Success. My favorite of all time is Og Mandino's *Keys to Success*, the audio version of his 15-million copy best-seller, *The Greatest Salesman in the World*, a phenomenal book for salespeople in all walks of life (in other words, for anyone).

Log on at www.truestarhealth.com for more information about the Truestar Daily Motivational Plan.

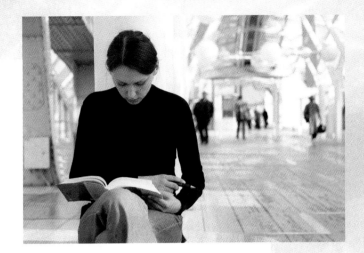

ATTITUDE AIDS

Top 10 Motivational Audio Tapes

1. *The Seven Spiritual Laws of Success* by Deepak Chopra
2. *The Greatest Salesman in the World (Keys to Success)* by Og Mandino
3. *Get The Edge* by Anthony Robbins
4. *How to Stay Motivated-Volume 1* by Zig Ziglar
5. *Raising Positive Kids in a Negative World* by Zig Ziglar
6. *The 7 Habits of Highly Effective People* by Stephen Covey
7. *How to Stay Motivated-Volume 2* by Zig Ziglar
8. *Maximum Achievement* by Brian Tracy
9. *How to Stay Motivated-Volume 3* by Zig Ziglar
10. *Personal Power 2* by Anthony Robbins

Top 10 Motivational Books

1. *The Seven Spiritual Laws of Success* by Deepak Chopra
2. *The Greatest Salesman in the World* by Og Mandino
3. *The Monk Who Sold his Ferrari* by Robin Sharma
4. *It's Not About the Bike* by Lance Armstrong
5. *The 7 Habits of Highly Effective People* by Stephen Covey
6. *Ten Things I Learned From Bill Porter* by Shelly Brady
7. *How to Win Friends and Influence People* by Dale Carnegie
8. *Think and Grow Rich* by Napoleon Hill
9. *The Road Less Traveled* by Dr M. Scott Peck
10. *Man's Search for Meaning* by Dr Viktor Frankl

Log on at www.truestarhealth.com to order many of these motivational audios and books.

"I believe in myself; I can do anything I set my mind to; I'm powerful." Now say this over at least 5 times and put some body language into it at the same time (clench your fists and pump your arms).

6. Positive Self-Talk

Successful people are solution-oriented, whereas people who fail often are problem dwellers.

Do you talk to yourself? We all do! Even if we don't speak aloud to ourselves, every thought we have is a form of self-talk. When you ask yourself questions, do you ask discouraging questions or empowering questions? 'Why am I always messing up?' or 'How can I improve myself?' Many leading motivational speakers recommend speaking aloud to yourself in a positive manner. Repeating a positive statement aloud can create an extremely powerful feeling, both mentally and physically.

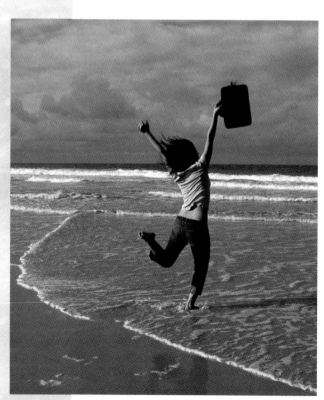

Incantations

Positive self-talk can be integrated into your life just as easily as gratitude rituals can be and also does not take a lot of time or money. It's very simple. Come up with a 3-step chant, such as, "I believe in myself; I can do anything I set my mind to; I'm powerful." Now say this over at least 5 times and put some body language into it at the same time (clench your fists and pump your arms). This technique is sure to lift you up and can be repeated over and over again during the day and even in silence if you're in a crowd and feel a little self-conscious about chanting out loud and pumping your arms.

Brian Tracy recommends repeating the phrase, "I like myself! I like myself! I like myself!" Zig Ziglar suggests standing in front of a mirror and reciting all your positive qualities, including qualities you want to acquire. Tony Robbins suggests finding powerful incantations to repeat aloud while simultaneously making a powerful physical action. Another incantation might be, "I'm strong, I'm a leader, I'm a helper of others!" We recommend finding a powerful incantation of your own to use on a daily basis to pick you up and put you over the top.

Log on to www.truestarhealth.com to create a personalized daily motivational plan.

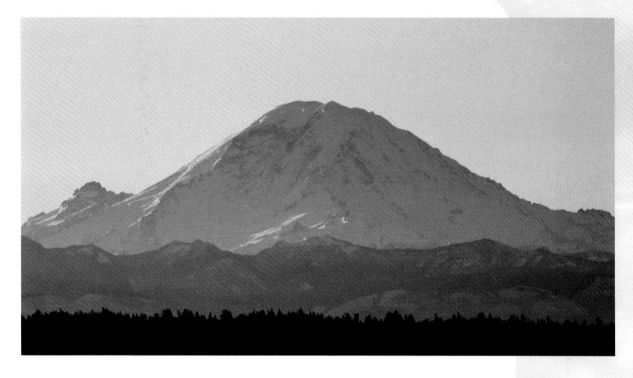

Fear of Failure

One of the major differences between success and failure is the way we talk to ourselves. As Tony Robbins says, "Failure is an event, not a person." So if you are using a failure's way of thinking and it's working, I suggest trying the exact opposite way of speaking to yourself.

- Successful people are solution-oriented, whereas people who fail often are problem dwellers.

- Successful people create reasons in their own mind to succeed, whereas people who fail often create reasons why they can't succeed.

I am personally extremely frightened of failure, which drives me to succeed. "People are motivated by two major feelings," Tony Robbins says, "which are pain and pleasure, and people will do more to avoid pain than to gain pleasure." This validates my contention that I'm so afraid to fail that I'll do almost anything to avoid it. The problem with many people is that fear of failure immobilizes and deters them from trying their hardest or even getting started on something, even though it may be a life dream, because they are afraid to fail.

> Successful people create reasons in their own mind to succeed, whereas people who fail often create reasons why they can't succeed.

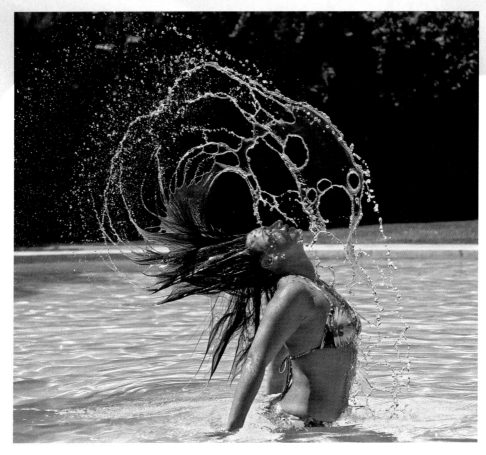

I'm a Tiger!

There are other ways to use positive self-talk to give yourself a boost in the short term or on a daily or hourly basis. My daughters play hockey, and their coach heard about the motivational program that I used with the Halton Hurricanes team. He asked me if I could help with his team — the Orangeville Tigers were on a long losing streak and he was getting desperate.

His request was music to my ears. I love motivating sports teams, and the idea of working with my daughter's team of 8-10 year old girls was exciting. I knew my program would have an impact because girls of that age tend to follow a program without much resistance. Most haven't started their rebellious years yet.

In addition to introducing goal-setting strategies to the team, we gave some tips on proper eating habits (which included a visit by Truestar's Dr Joey Shulman) and developed a positive self-talk program. The girls come up with a 3-step incantation or chant that they used all game long: "I believe in Myself, I'm a Tiger, and I'm Powerful !" When they chanted it out loud, they clenched their fists to create a physically powerful feeling with their body. They would chant all game long.

Soon the team started to improve. Two weeks after the program started, the Tigers won more than just a game — they won an entire tournament.

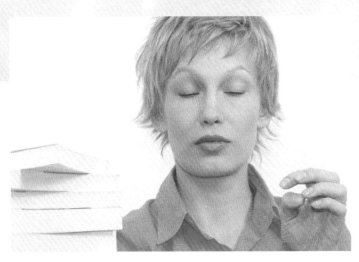

7. Visualization

Visualization goes hand in hand with goal setting because once you set your goal, your ability to see yourself reaching that goal clearly in your mind is paramount to success. Visualization is a skill used by all highly effective people, whether they are conscious of it or not. It is simply a technique of focusing in a highly concentrated manner on a task, project, or goal. Visualization has been used by highly successful athletes, such as Michael Jordan, Jack Nicklaus, and Wayne Gretzky, as well as by neurosurgeons and successful business executives. Maxwell Maltz's book, *Visualization*, has been used by many Fortune 500 companies in training their executives and salespeople.

To accelerate the rate of achieving your goals, daily tasks, or projects, visualize in a highly focused and concentrated manner on your desired results. For high-level tasks, such as athletic performances, public speaking, or sales presentations, visualization should be done for hours to prepare for the very best outcome. For less intense but important issues, such as day-to-day interactions, visualization can improve outcomes dramatically. You should spend at least one hour each day visualizing the achievement of your goals and how you will achieve them. Visualization is a key tool in nurturing a positive, thriving attitude.

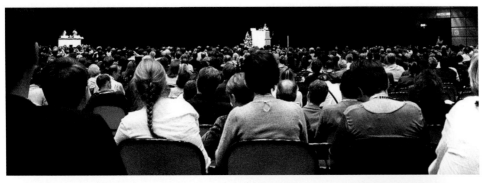

Shooting Baskets

One well-known study on visualization was done using three groups of 10 prison inmates who were asked to shoot basketball free throws. The first group was allowed to practice free throws for one week. The second group was not allowed to practice and was not told a study was being done. The third group was told there was a study being done and was asked to visualize shooting free throws for the next week. After the week-long practice and visualization period, the three groups were asked to shoot 10 free throws per person. The first group, which had been practicing, shot with over 80% accuracy. The second group, which was not informed about the study and had not practiced, shot with just over 30% accuracy. The third group, which had been visualizing all week long but not physically practicing, ended up shooting 73% or more than double the group that had not visualized.

ATTITUDE AIDS FOR VISUALIZATION
- *Visualization* by Maxwell Maltz
- *Maximum Achievement* by Brian Tracy

8. Relaxing and Winding Down

Find a quiet place in your home where you can spend 15 minutes each day in solitude.

Some people have trouble getting wound up, excited, or passionate about their lives. Other so-called type A personalities have difficulty winding down. This can lead to poor sleep, hypertension, and strained relationships.

In his best-selling motivational fable, *The Monk Who Sold His Ferrari*, Robin Sharma recommends finding a quiet place in your home where you can spend 15 minutes each day in solitude to help keep yourself in balance. Mahatma Gandhi, one of the greatest leaders in the 20th century, would spend Sunday evening until Monday evening each week in complete solitude and silence to regroup and refocus for the week ahead. Deepak Chopra calls this silent time "getting in touch with self." Some people may consider this practice a waste of time, but Gandhi proved to the world that his time for self allowed him to be more effective in one week than some of us may be in one month or even one year!

ATTITUDE AIDS FOR RELAXATION
- *The Seven Spiritual Laws of Success* by Deepak Chopra Sharma,
- *The Monk Who Sold His Ferrari* by Robin Sharma
- www.mkganhdi.org/index.htm

9. Reducing TV and News

Dr Andrew Weil recommends a "news fast" as a step toward improved health in his book *8 Weeks to Optimum Health*. Listening to or reading the news once or more a day can often be disturbing to the conscious and subconscious mind. Not only are many world events very disturbing, television programs accentuate the negative, driven by ratings to provide shock value. Not very often when you turn on news or read the papers do you hear about good deeds.

How does disturbing news and sensational programming affect our personal attitude, our relationships, actions, and outcomes? Is the news helping me or hurting me?

While it may be important to be informed about world events, how much control do you have over these world events? Will watching disturbing information before going to bed disturb your sleep? Will it have a subconscious and real affect on you?

Taking a break from negative, sensational, or useless information allows you to control your input. Try reading a book as a substitute for television watching and try your own news fast. The result may be a happier, calmer, more focused you.

ATTITUDE AIDS
- *8 Weeks to Optimum Health* by Andrew Weil

10. Giving

Have you ever noticed how excited grandparents are to see their grandchild? It may be that as we grow older, we finally realize that the true path to happiness is giving. Grandparents are excited because of the opportunity to give to their grandchild, whether the gift is a present, a nice meal, or simply the gift of time or love.

Are you more excited giving a gift or receiving one? Deepak Chopra refers to "The Law of Giving and Receiving": when we give unconditionally, our giving will come back to us as part of the constant flow of life's abundance. Start giving today, whether your gift is material, verbal or even a thought!

ATTITUDE AIDS FOR GIVING
- *The Seven Spiritual Laws of Success* by Deepak Chopra
- *The Greatest Salesman in the World* by Og Mandino

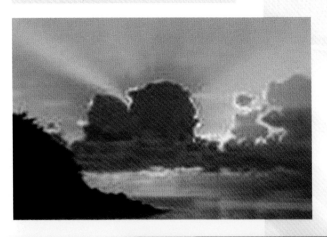

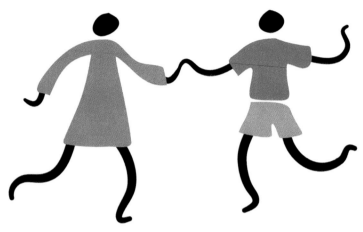

11. Remaining Non-Judgmental

Not only do we need to cultivate an attitude of being non-judgmental in our relations with other people, we need to be non-judgmental with ourselves.

Being judgmental is another negative attitude that will stifle personal growth. We become close-minded, no longer open to change. Remaining non-judgmental, however, is one of the most difficult positive attitude traits, yet perhaps one of the most effective. When I first read about being non-judgmental in Deepak Chopra's book *The Seven Spiritual Laws of Success*, the idea made perfect sense for developing a positive attitude. Being non-judgmental doesn't mean that you're going to condone what everyone else is doing or adopt every new trend or habit that comes along. It does mean that you won't judge prematurely or summarily and will keep an open mind — unless of course someone is committing a crime or may hurt another person.

For me, being non-judgmental can be difficult when I'm evaluating an employee's job performance and growth. The secret to being non-judgmental in these situations is to realize that failure or success is an event, not a person. Because I focus on the performance, not the person, I've given my employees a better chance of developing than others might have. By not being judgmental, I think that I've helped many employees become successful people.

Not only do we need to cultivate an attitude of being non-judgmental in our relations with other people, we need to be non-judgmental with ourselves. If you're like me and you're very hard on yourself when you make a mistake, you could be affecting your health. As time has gone by, I've become less hard on myself. I find there is an associated calmness in doing so.

ATTITUDE AIDS FOR REMAINING NON-JUDGMENTAL
□ *The Seven Spiritual Laws of Success* by Deepak Chopra

> "The greatest danger for most of us is not that we aim too high and we miss it,
> but we aim too low and we reach it." Michelangelo

12. Monitoring Positive Attitude

"A negative thought," Anthony Robbins says, "is a signal that something has to change." When you are feeling negative, consider what changes need to be made to accentuate the positive. Negative thoughts can also simply be "FEAR, represented as 'False Evidence Appearing Real'," Robbins says. Try to dispel the false evidence by looking more closely at the cause of your fear. We often attach the intense emotion of fear to something that we shouldn't be obsessing about at all. Fear is a state of mind. Feeling negative is, too. Being optimistic that the outcome will be positive regardless will eliminate many unnecessary fears.

When you experience negative thoughts, think back to your morning gratitude ritual, and remember all that you have to be thankful for. It may help if you write down your morning gratitude thoughts so you can refer to them throughout the day. You can also take positive action in the form of positive body language and full, deep breathing. "Action makes you positive," Anthony Robbins says, "and inaction makes you negative." Monitor your attitude and be sure it isn't slipping. A poor attitude can lead to poor decision-making — even to poor health.

ATTITUDE AIDS FOR MONITORING A POSITIVE ATTITUDE
- *The Seven Spiritual Laws of Success* by Deepak Chopra
- *Personal Power 2* by Anthony Robbins
- *Get the Edge* by Anthony Robbins
- *How to Stay Motivated Volume 1 — Developing the Qualities of Success* by Zig Ziglar

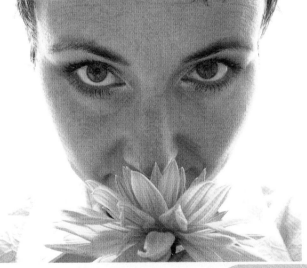

When you experience negative thoughts, think back to your morning gratitude ritual, and remember all that you have to be thankful for.

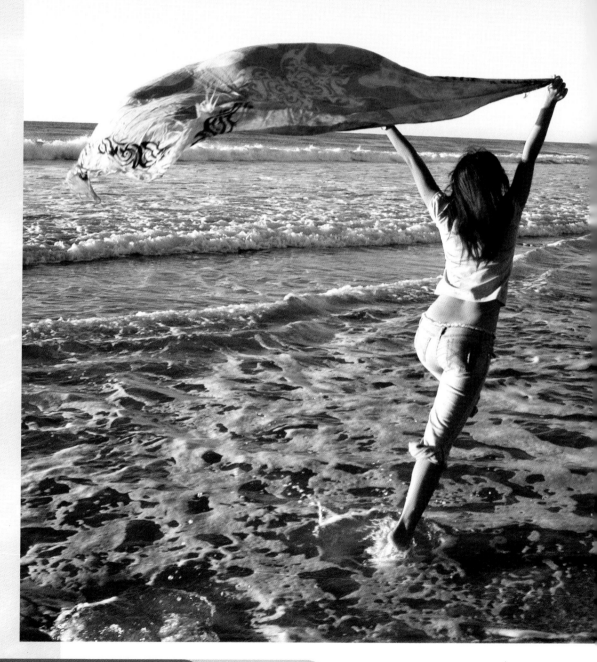

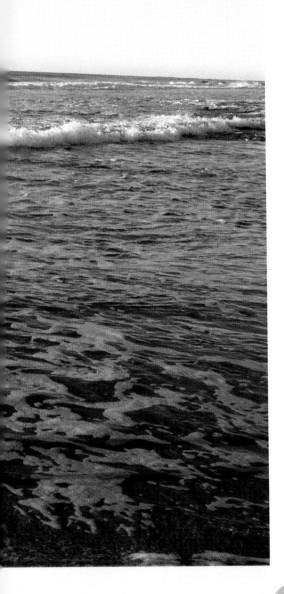

The Truestar Way …

So, there you have it, the Truestar way to good attitude. Every day situations arise that will test success habits. These challenging situations require positive and controlled actions. You may not be able to control every situation, but you can control how you react to the situation by following the Truestar life improvement program.

When you combine a positive attitude with good nutrition, regular exercise, and vitamin supplements, you are well on your way to total health and weight loss. Now, just add some good sleep habits … and your goal will be within reach.

You may not be able to control every situation, but you can control how you react to the situation by following the Truestar Life Improvement Program.

Sleep

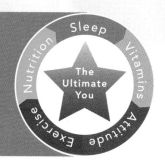

Ah, Sleep!

Tim Mulcahy

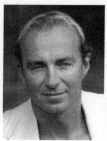

Tim Mulcahy

Sleep Country, a company that sells beds, advertises that 88% of the population is sleep deprived. I'm sure that many of us find ourselves in this state some of the time, a few of us, all of the time. Poor sleep can lead to serious health disorders, while good sleep can prevent illness.

As my life continues to unfold, sleep is the one area of Truestar's five principles of total health that I continue to work on. While I now eat nutritious meals, exercise regularly, take my vitamins, and work hard on maintaining a positive attitude, I don't always sleep well. However, after recently getting some sleep tips from Dr Natasha Turner, one of Truestar's staff experts, I've improved my sleep habits significantly. Just little changes can have a really positive impact.

Improving my overall sleep habits remains one of my goals. I know how great I feel when I do get a good night's sleep (I feel my best at 7 to 9 hours). I achieve this about three or four nights out of seven and would like to increase that to seven out of seven. One of the problems I have is winding down. Sometimes I will fall asleep at 11:00, but then wake up at 3:00 and can't get back to sleep because my mind engages and won't shut down. I used to fight this and try desperately to get back to sleep, losing sleep over losing sleep. Now, I realize that I may be awake because I do have a lot to think about. I may not have had much time to think during the day because I was too busy. I've given up the fight to get back to sleep. Staying awake thinking is not as draining as becoming anxious over my sleep loss.

There's no question that lack of sleep is hard to overcome; however, I find that if I eat less during the day after not having enough sleep, as well as get in a light workout, take my vitamins, and remain positive, I can still function at close to 100%. Even so, a committed regimen of good sleep habits is the ideal.

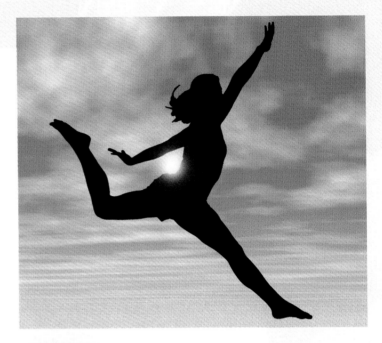

Here are some benefits of getting a good night's sleep:

- You will awaken feeling refreshed
- You will be more creative and have improved concentration
- You will feel more positive
- Your relationships with others will improve
- Your sex drive will return or improve
- You will be calmer and more alert throughout the day
- You may lose weight permanently and safely
- You will be happier — and isn't that the point of it all?

Excuse me while I turn in and enjoy some of these benefits.

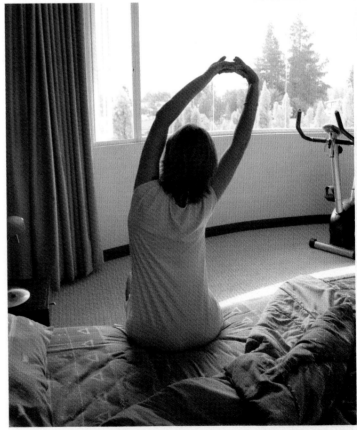

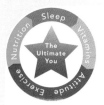

Sleep... the Truestar Way

Dr Natasha Turner, ND
Vice-President, Natural Medicine

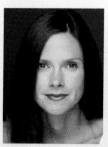

Natasha Turner

Because of the increasingly hectic pace of our lives, we have become more sleep deprived than ever before. Many of us spend a great deal of time at our jobs, driven by deadlines and quotas, while trying to balance time with our family and keeping up with our personal relationships. We are exposed to a steady stream of stimulation from televisions, radios, computers, and telephones.

Our diets are full of sugar, caffeine, and processed foods. We rarely get enough physical activity, fresh air, or sunshine. We don't get up and go to bed following the regular cycle of the sun the way our ancestors did. We are exposed to artificial light 24 hours a day. Since the invention of electricity, we have begun to stay up later and later.

All of these behaviors have contributed to a high incidence of chronic sleep deprivation and sleep disorders. Fortunately, healthy sleep patterns can be re-established by re-educating our minds and bodies — the Truestar way.

We all know sleep is required for our body to repair and rejuvenate. Rebuilding our reserves nightly enables us to take on each new day with enthusiasm and helps us to adapt more easily to the stresses of daily life. Think of how anxieties seem to build the later we stay up or how much better things can seem in the morning after a good night's sleep. Simply making an effort to improve your sleep habits can enhance your quality of life and give you the energy you need to be successful in your pursuits. Who knows — as you will soon discover — you may be able to sleep yourself thin ...

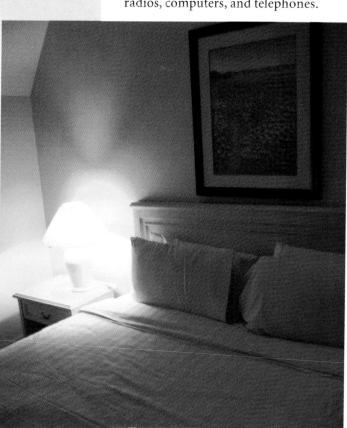

A-ZZZs of Sleep

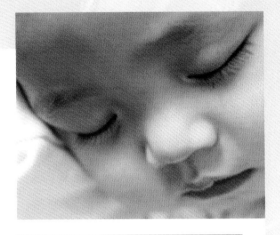

Sleep Cycles

There are five cycles of sleep: Stage 1 to 3 are light sleep, Stage 4 is very deep sleep, and Stage 5 is REM (rapid eye movement) sleep. Stages 1 to 4 are commonly grouped together and called non-REM sleep.

The majority of sleep, greater than 50%, occurs in the fourth cycle, deep sleep, while we spend about 20% to 25% of our sleep time in the REM cycle. The two sleep states, non-REM and REM, alternate between 90 and 110 minute intervals throughout the night. Early in the evening, the deep sleep periods are longer, sometimes up to an hour, whereas REM periods typically last only a few minutes. Later in the night, the deep sleep phases are shorter and REM periods lengthen. This pattern causes us to dream during the second half of the night.

During REM sleep, we dream and our brain activity is similar to waking state activity. Interestingly, our limbs become paralyzed during REM sleep to prevent us from acting out our dreams, but there is a sleep disorder where this paralyzation of limbs does not happen. REM sleep is essential to good health. A deficiency has been linked to fatigue, moodiness, irritability, and depression.

Sleep Medication Alert

Some sleep medications may actually result in REM-deficient sleep, which can leave many users waking up feeling unrefreshed. Because REM sleep is found to be lacking with sleep aids, it is suggested these types of medications may shorten our life span if used long-term.

The Purpose of Sleep

Simply stated, if we have enough sleep, we feel and perform better, but there are many other reasons why sleep is important for health.

Restorative

Sleep enables the body and mind to rejuvenate, re-energize, and restore. It is believed that as a person sleeps, the brain reorganizes and integrates new information and memories. Tissues, nerve cells, and certain hormone levels undergo a process of repair and renewal in response to hormonal changes during sleep. Sleep allows the body to recuperate and the mind to sort out past, present, and future actions and feelings.

Simply making an effort to improve your sleep habits can enhance your quality of life and give you the energy you need to be successful in your pursuits. Who knows, soon you may be able to sleep yourself thin ...

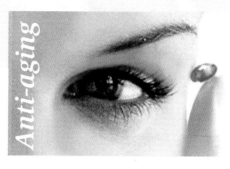
Programming

Some researchers postulate the brain filters information while we sleep during the REM stage. Unimportant information is erased, while important information is stored for future access. This occurrence of mental activity during sleep may explain why there are higher levels of REM sleep in students and others who complete intellectual activities during the day.

Growth and Development

Human growth hormone is released in children and adults during deep sleep. This hormone orchestrates the process of repair and helps rebuild lean body mass and bone. Without enough sleep, your body will not repair as effectively and may age prematurely as a result. Many of the body's cells also show increased production and reduced breakdown of proteins during deep

Deep sleep
may truly be
beauty sleep.

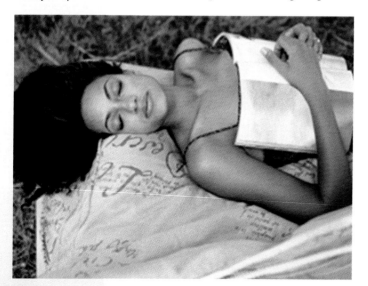

sleep. Since proteins are the building blocks needed for cell growth and the repair of damage caused by such factors as stress and ultraviolet rays, deep sleep may truly be *beauty sleep.*

Anti-Aging

Watching the late show every night? Putting TV ahead of your sleep may be affecting more than just your energy and productivity the next day. Your current sleep habits are unknowingly causing you to age at an accelerated rate — metabolically and physically. Even worse, many of us who choose to stay up and trade off sleep for other activities eventually adapt and feel less fatigued. Regularly following these poor sleep habits puts you in a metabolic state that is commonly found in seniors!

Immune Function

Sleep restores your immune system and helps it to function properly, making you less susceptible to colds, flu, and infection. Researchers at Penn State University and the National Institute of Health Child Health and Human Development group found a relationship between a lack of sleep and the impairment of day-to-day functions, as well as elevated immune hormones in healthy men and women similar to when fighting an infection.

Flu Fighters

Infectious diseases, like the flu, tend to make us feel sleepy. This likely occurs because cytokines, chemicals our immune system produces while fighting infection or inflammation, are powerful sleep-inducing agents. Sleep may help the body conserve energy and other resources the immune system needs to mount an attack against bacterial or viral invaders. Stages 3 and 4 of sleep are most important for restoration.

Recuperation from Stress

Sleep aids in the prevention of stress-induced disorders, such as depression, fatigue, and anxiety.

Fat Burning

The optimal time for fat burning occurs between your evening meal and breakfast. Try to avoid eating after 8 p.m. and ensure the fasting period lasts for at least 11 hours to achieve maximum fat burning. The release of growth hormone and reduction of insulin levels in the absence of food and snacks creates the perfect hormonal balance for fat burning while you sleep, provided you try to go to bed by 10 p.m.

New research suggests a reduction in the number of hours slept can cause an increase in the release of the stress hormone cortisol. Cortisol affects appetite and may cause some people to feel hungry even when they have consumed

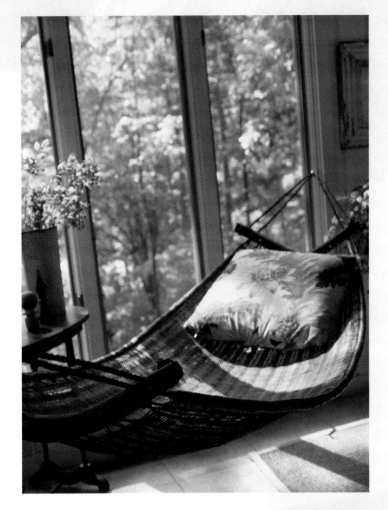

appropriate amounts of food.

Inadequate sleep may also cause abnormalities in blood sugar regulation, resulting in high blood glucose levels, which then stimulates high insulin levels. Insulin is a hormone which, when present, allows sugars to enter cells to be used as fuel. If the fuel is not burned, it is stored as fat. It is unlikely that any of this sugar will be used as fuel during sleep, so this can lead to an increase in body fat. The long-term effect of this pattern is insulin resistance, a predisposing factor to type II or adult onset diabetes .

Try to avoid eating after 8 p.m. and ensure the fasting period lasts for at least 11 hours to achieve maximum fat burning.

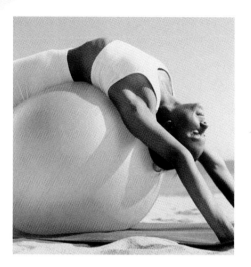

What Makes Us Sleep?

Years ago, it was believed our brains would literally tire out, causing us to go to sleep. However, an important experiment that purposely damaged areas of the brain showed that the brain never sleeps! This suggested there is actually an area of the brain that makes us sleep and another that keeps us alert. When certain areas of the brain remain active for periods of time, they fatigue, and then other areas of the brain that regulate sleep become activated. This means that sleep is, in fact, an active process, not passive.

Through a complex process of hormonal and neurological changes, daylight naturally triggers periods of wakefulness. The longer a person stays awake, the more sleep required; thus, the need to sleep accumulates throughout the time of wakefulness. This maintains a balance as it allows the body to reverse the effects of sleepiness by sleeping, helping to prevent slept debt.

Circadian Rhythm

The natural rhythm of being awake and being asleep is a circadian or daily rhythm in our lives. Sleepy times or 'peaks' naturally occur every 12 hours for most people, around mid-afternoon and at night, usually between 3:00 and 4:00 a.m. The sleepy peak in the mid afternoon most often corresponds to the time after lunch. After eating, the body temperature drops. A drop in body temperature makes us sleepier than when it is steady or rising.

One of the many functions of our brain is to regulate our internal environment to maintain a steady state or homeostasis. It is influenced by a structure in the brain called the hypothalamus. Homeostasis is involved in the natural pattern of our sleep and wakefulness.

SCN REGULATION

The hypothalamus is divided into several sections or nuclei. The suprachiasmatic nuclei (SCN) regulate our internal clock or circadian rhythm. Our circadian rhythm, controlled by the light sensitive SCN, closely regulates the reasons why we need to sleep. Studies have shown that the absence of light does not disable our biological clocks, but, without time cues, it seems to normalize to 25 hours instead of 24. However, the sensitivity of the SCN to light may explain why daytime resting is not as effective as nighttime sleep.

The SCN governs functions that are synchronized with the sleep/wake cycle, including body temperature, hormone secretion, urine production, and changes in blood pressure. Body temperature is directly linked to our level of arousal; the warmer we are the more alert we become. This explains why cooling down after a hot shower induces sleep.

MELATONIN

Signals from the SCN travel to several brain regions, including the pineal gland, which responds to light-induced signals by switching off production of the hormone melatonin. The body's level of melatonin normally increases after darkness falls, making people feel drowsy. Because melatonin is a powerful antioxidant, it aids in turning on the nighttime repair processes. Melatonin production is suppressed when you are in the light — even the small amount of light from a digital alarm clock can affect its release. Therefore, it is best to keep your bedroom pitch black for sleeping.

SEROTONIN

Serotonin is another brain chemical (a neurotransmitter) involved in the process of sleep. When animals are given drugs to inhibit the release of serotonin, they do not sleep for days. Many of the sleeping pills given today affect serotonin release and production; however, the complete role of serotonin in sleep is confusing because serotonin levels are actually lower in the blood during sleep than during the day. This suggests that there are other hormones involved in the regulation of healthy sleep patterns. In REM sleep, serotonin levels drop almost to zero, allowing it to be preserved for later daily use. Individuals lacking REM sleep usually have lower levels of serotonin in conjunction with conditions like depression or anxiety.

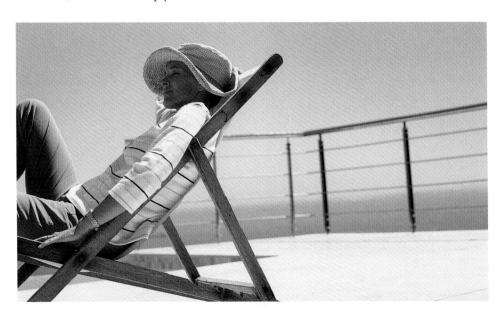

It is best to keep your bedroom pitch black for sleeping.

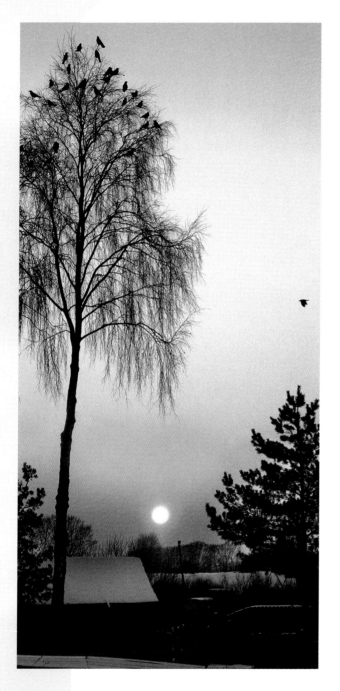

Psychological Mechanisms

Sleep has effects on the nervous system, as well as on other structures in the body. During sleep, sympathetic nervous system stimulation decreases, while parasympathetic stimulation increases. These two nervous systems regulate the fight or flight response. The sympathetic response stimulation occurs during a fight-like situation, while parasympathetic stimulation is activated when we are in 'couch potato' mode. During wakefulness, there is more sympathetic nervous system stimulation as well as more nerve signals to the skeletal muscles to enhance muscle tone. During restful sleep, parasympathetic stimulation is highest, blood pressure falls, pulse rate decreases, skin blood vessels dilate, muscles relax, the metabolic rate usually falls by 10% to 30%, and sometimes the activity of the intestines increases.

Sleep Debt

This gives you some idea of what happens when you don't get enough sleep. Students, medical residents, executives, workaholics, shift workers, new parents, and most of the remaining population create sleep debt when their personal requirements for sleep are not met.

Daytime drowsiness or the desire to sleep later is the body's natural reaction to a lack of sleep. Keep in mind that many

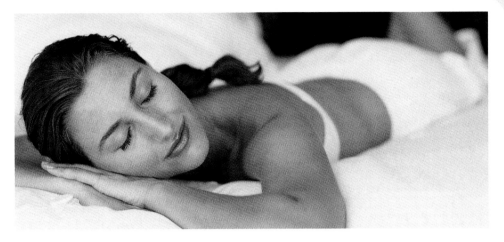

of us are extremely poor judges of our own fatigue levels and most likely require more rest than we may allow ourselves.

Repaying sleep debt requires more sleep than usual. In most cases, though, sleep debt has a natural way of resolving itself because the relationship between wakefulness and sleep discourages us from becoming dangerously sleep deprived. The natural active process the brain undergoes to ensure sleep helps to maintain natural sleep patterns even when we may overwork.

Sleep Deprived?

If you answer "yes" to the following questions, you are probably sleep deprived.

- ☐ Do you fall asleep as soon as your head hits the pillow?
- ☐ Do you wake with an alarm?
- ☐ Do you fail to wake up just a few moments before your alarm goes off?
- ☐ Do you feel tired during the day?
- ☐ Do you sleep more on the weekends?

Health Consequences

Performance
Studies have shown that without enough sleep, a person's ability to perform even simple tasks declines significantly. The average sleep-deprived individual may experience impaired performance, lack of concentration, and daytime drowsiness. They are less alert and attentive, unable to concentrate effectively.

Emotional Well-Being
Persistent sleep deprivation can cause significant mood swings, irritability, erratic behavior, hallucinations, and, in extremely rare cases, death. Activity in the parts of the brain that controls emotions, decision-making processes, and social interactions is drastically reduced during deep sleep. This suggests that deep sleep may help people maintain optimal emotional and social functioning while they are awake.

Keep in mind that many of us are extremely poor judges of our own fatigue levels and most likely require more rest than we may allow ourselves.

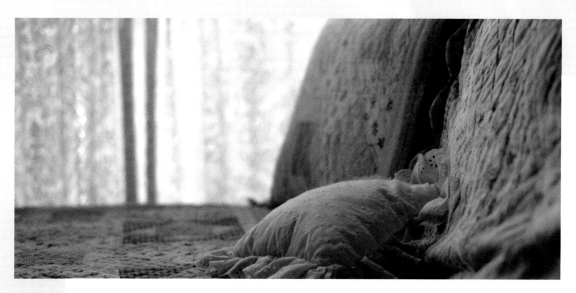

How Much Sleep Is Enough?

The optimal amount of sleep is 7 to 9 hours per night, in pitch black, ideally with going to bed before 11 p.m. The American Cancer Association found higher incidences of cancer in individuals who consistently slept 6 hours or less or more than 9 hours nightly. New research recently reported that individuals who regularly slept 7 hours per night lived longer. However, some people may require more or less than others. If you wake without an alarm and you feel refreshed upon rising, you are most likely getting enough sleep for you. As for teenagers, they are not just lazy after all. They require more sleep — around 9½ hours nightly.

Diabetes and Heart Disease

Lower rates of diabetes and heart disease are associated with adequate rest and recuperation. Studies have found that higher levels of glucose intolerance, a pre-diabetic condition, are associated with sleep deprivation.

Mental Disorders

Sleeping problems occur in almost all people with mental disorders, including those with depression, anxiety, manic depression, and schizophrenia. In addition, sleep deprivation may actually cause or contribute to depression or anxiety disorders, making it difficult to determine which came first.

People with depression or anxiety often wake up in the early hours of the morning or soon after going to bed and find themselves unable to get back to sleep. The amount of sleep a person gets also strongly influences the symptoms of mental disorders.

Sleep deprivation can be an effective therapy for people with certain types of depression associated with a tendency to oversleep, while it can actually cause depression in others who have insomnia associated with depression. Extreme sleep deprivation can lead to a seemingly psychotic state of paranoia and hallucination in otherwise healthy people, and disrupted sleep can trigger episodes of mania (agitation and hyperactivity) in people with manic depression.

Epilepsy

Sleep affects some kinds of epilepsy in complex ways. REM sleep seems to help prevent seizures that begin in one part of the brain from spreading to other brain regions, while deep sleep may promote the spread of these seizures. Sleep deprivation also triggers seizures in people with some types of epilepsy.

Pain Management

Patients who are experiencing pain and are unable to sleep may notice their pain more and increase their requests for pain medication. The interaction between sleep and pain is important in patients suffering from arthritis, fibromyalgia, and other chronic pain conditions. Not only can pain disturb sleep, but alterations in the deeper sleep stages, induced by pain and inflammation, may also decrease the pain threshold, as well as the ability to heal, because growth hormone, important for rebuilding body tissues, is reduced.

Sleep Disorders

Snoring and Sleep Apnea

Individuals who have a sleep disorder called sleep apnea or who snore have increased risks of being pre-diabetic (insulin resistant), experiencing full-blown type II diabetes, or suffering cardiovascular disease.

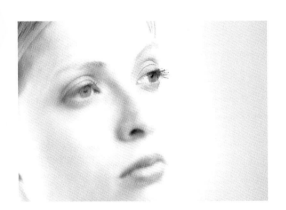

Sleep apnea is an obstructive disorder characterized by repeated episodes of partial or complete cessation of breathing during sleep. Apneas are considered clinically significant if they last at least 10 seconds, although they usually last for 20 to 30 seconds and may exceed a full minute.

Types of Sleep Apnea

Obstructive apnea is the absence of airflow despite an effort to breathe. Central apnea is the absence of airflow due to a lack of ventilatory effort. Mixed apnea begins with the central component of effortless breathing, followed by a lack of airflow, despite the fact the patient is trying to breathe.

The amount of sleep a person gets also strongly influences the symptoms of mental disorders. Sleep deprivation may actually cause or contribute to depression or anxiety disorders, making it difficult to determine which came first.

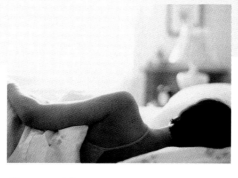

Signs and Symptoms

Sleep apnea is characterized by snoring, daytime sleepiness, repeated interruptions of breathing during sleep (either partial or complete), arousal from sleep, and possibly morning headaches. Long-term sufferers may experience symptoms of fatigue, mood swings, obesity, low sex drive, and poor concentration.

Individuals who snore or have sleep apnea may be unaware of their condition. They may deny or minimize their sleep-disordered breathing because of embarrassment. A family member or life-partner may be need to report snoring or sleep apnea to the individual or to their healthcare professional.

The mechanism for the association of diabetes and insulin resistance with sleep apnea has not yet been determined but one could postulate it may be related to an elevation of stress hormones while sleeping, with disrupted air flow.

WEIGHT GAIN

This condition is more common in overweight or obese individuals and has been linked to high blood pressure, increased risk of heart attack and stroke, diabetes, and insulin resistance, which causes a compensatory increase in the amount of insulin produced by the pancreas. High levels of insulin are associated with increased abdominal fat, especially in the 'love handles' area, as well as high blood triglyceride levels. Excess carbohydrate intake causes a further elevation of insulin, which then causes more weight gain. As well, symptoms of blood sugar irregularities, such as sleepiness after meals, increased hunger, weakness, irritability, dizziness or fatigue, which may result without frequent snacking, tend to be associated with insulin resistance.

Causes

Most sleep apnea episodes are caused by a collapse of the throat airway. During sleep, muscle tone relaxes and may result in a narrowing of the upper airway during inhalation, resulting in snoring. The airway narrowing also leads to an increased respiratory effort and arousal. The arousal restores the muscle tone of the upper airways, allowing the individual to fall asleep once again. In sleep apnea, the cycle of sleep and arousal may be repeated throughout the night. Substances that relax muscles, such as alcohol and tranquilizers (benzodiazepines), tend to exacerbate sleep apnea.

Diagnosis

The best way to determine if you are experiencing sleep apnea is to speak to your doctor, who can then refer you for a sleep study. You should also ask your family members if they notice breathing disruption while you sleep.

High levels of insulin are associated with increased abdominal fat, especially in the 'love handles' area, as well as high blood triglyceride levels.

Log on to www.truestarhealth.com for more information on preventive strategies for sleep disorders.

Sleep Apnea Treatments

☐ CPAP: Sleep apnea may be treated with continuous positive airway pressure (CPAP), which maintains the patency of the upper respiratory airways during sleep. CPAP is a small air compressor and a mask worn during the night to ensure that the sleeper continues to breathe. Although the long-term effects are unclear, treatment of sleep apnea by CPAP was shown to decrease blood pressure acutely during sleep. While CPAP is the definitive treatment, it may be poorly tolerated by patients.

☐ ORAL DEVICES: Another non-surgical method of treatment is the use of oral devices that change the position of the jaws and tongue during sleep.

☐ UPPP: As a final resort, sleep apnea may be treated with surgery. Uvulopalatopharngoplasty (UPPP) reshapes the uvula and soft palate by removing excess tissue from the throat area of sleep apnea patients.

The Truestar Way

Because of the close association between body weight, diabetes risk, and sleep apnea, the Truestar nutrition plan is perfect for anyone with sleep apnea. For those at risk of diabetes, our Truestar supplement plan for healthy blood sugar balance is a must. Finally, for risk associated with cardio-vascular health, our Truestar supplement plan for heart health provides good preventive measures and may assist with a current heart condition, including high cholesterol and high blood pressure. Your supplement plan, used in conjunction with your Truestar dietary and exercise plan, will result in a significant reduction in risk for type II diabetes and heart disease, as well as a reduction in the symptoms or severity of sleep apnea or snoring. Exercise is essential for reducing blood pressure, improving your body's response to insulin, and maintaining a healthy body weight.

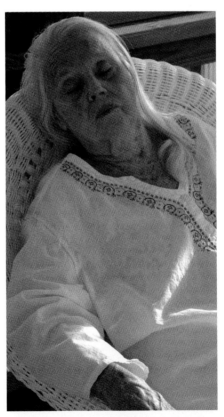

Substances that relax muscles, such as alcohol and tranquilizers (benzodiazepines), tend to exacerbate sleep apnea.

Night Eating Syndrome

Skip breakfast because you just don't feel like eating? Not hungry at lunch so you grab a muffin? By the end of the day you've consumed very few calories. Then at 8:00 p.m., when most people have finished eating for the day, you are standing in front of the fridge door eating everything in sight.

This is not a diet consistent with the hormonally balanced Truestar nutrition plan. Rather, this pattern of low caloric intake during the day, with over 50% of calories ingested in the evening, and waking up at least once a night amid intense food cravings, chiefly for carbohydrates, is characteristic of night eating syndrome (NES).

NES, a relatively uncommon condition, was originally thought to be a sleep disorder because it is often associated with insomnia. However, the tendency to binge in the evening is typical of an eating disorder. Currently, it's estimated that between 1% and 2% of adults may have night eating syndrome, yet it is postulated it may occur in up to 4% of obese people.

There is no doubt that NES can be an obstacle for weight loss and result in decreased vitality. However, the proper supplements, eating habits, sleep hygiene, and exercise program, as well as natural hormone assistance, can provide relief.

Causes

The delicate balance of the hormones involved with healthy sleep, response to stress, and appetite regulation is at the root of NES.

Currently, it's estimated that between 1% and 2% of adults may have night eating syndrome, yet it is postulated it may occur in up to 4% of obese people.

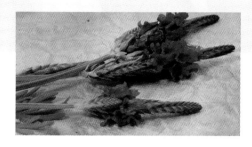

LOW MELATONIN: Not surprisingly, many cases of NES have been found to be associated with low levels of melatonin. Melatonin is necessary for healthy sleep patterns, including falling and staying asleep. Melatonin is reduced if we eat too close to bedtime. If melatonin does not get released, its cooling effect on body temperature necessary to induce sleep does not occur.

INCREASED CORTISOL: Cortisol is a stimulating hormone released when we are under stress. It is naturally highest around 6:00 a.m. in preparation for the day, gradually decreases throughout the day and evening, and peaks slightly at 2:00 a.m. and 4:00 a.m. as it begins to increase to its highest level again. Most individuals who are sleep deprived have abnormally high levels of cortisol in the evening and during the day. It is also found to be elevated in people with NES. High levels of cortisol in the evening may result in an inability to fall asleep, leading to more eating, as well as a pattern of waking between 2:00 and 4:00 a.m., characteristic of stress.

LOW LEPTIN: Leptin is the chemical signal that tells us we are full and keeps our appetite in check. Leptin was not found to rise to normal levels during sleep in NES sufferers, which may account for the sleep disturbing hunger pangs.

Night Eating Syndrome Treatments

An effective treatment plan for NES must involve a multifaceted approach directed at raising melatonin levels, managing stress, and assisting in weight loss. Along with the dietary habits in the Truestar weight loss program, the following are also of benefit:

RELORA: Preferably taken in the evening, relora has been found to reduce high cortisol levels, as well as aid in weight loss around the abdomen. It is also useful to assist with re-establishing healthy sleep patterns. *Dose:* 600 mg per day

5-HTP: Best taken in the evening, 5-HTP is an excellent means to increase serotonin levels, deficiencies of which have been linked to insomnia, over-consumption of carbohydrates, and stress-related eating. TrueCRAVE contains 5-HTP and other nutrients to reduce cravings for sugar and carbohydrates. *Dose:* 50-200 mg per day

MELATONIN: Since the majority of people with NES have low levels of melatonin, it only seems rational that supplements of it may provide benefit. *Dose:* 3 mg pill, taken nightly, in conjunction with the two products above, is useful in many cases

EXERCISE: Exercise in the morning will help to reduce cortisol levels, as well as aid weight loss. See the Truestar exercise section for your personalized exercise plan.

High levels of cortisol in the evening may result in an inability to fall asleep, leading to more eating, as well as a pattern of waking between 2:00 and 4:00 a.m., which is characteristic of stress.

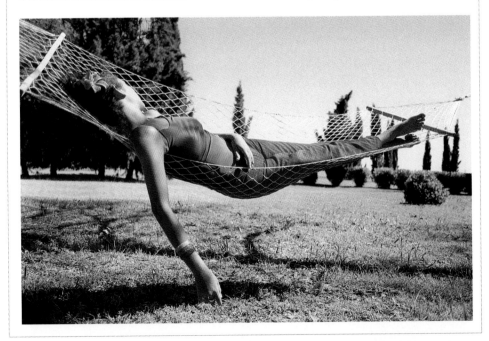

Insomnia

Generally speaking, insomnia is defined as poor-quality, inadequate, or insufficient sleep. It can be due to difficulty falling asleep, broken sleep due to frequently waking, waking in the middle of the night or early morning with difficulty returning to sleep, or simply related to unrefreshing sleep. Insomnia is not defined by the number of hours of sleep a person gets, but sometimes by how long it takes to fall asleep. Greater than 45 minutes to an hour after going to bed is the benchmark. Regardless of the sleep disruption pattern associated with insomnia, the end result is problematic daytime fatigue, poor concentration, a lack of energy and motivation, low immunity, accelerated aging, and irritability.

> Insomnia is not defined by the number of hours of sleep a person gets, but sometimes by how long it takes to fall asleep. Greater than 45 minutes to an hour after going to bed is the benchmark.

Types of Insomnia
- Transient insomnia (a few days)
- Intermittent insomnia (on and off over a period of time)
- Chronic insomnia (most nights, lasting more than a month)

The stress of work deadlines, family issues, a nasty break up, or other life upsets have caused the occasional sleepless night for many of us. But it is important to recognize recurrent or chronic insomnia because either may be an indication of an underlying medical condition or behavior related to sleeplessness.

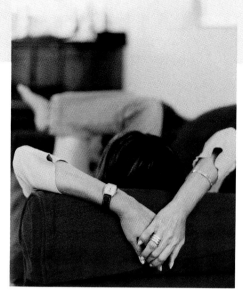

Causes of Insomnia and Sleep Disruption

Natural Causes
- Aging (insomnia is more frequent in individuals over 60)
- Women (females tend to have insomnia more often than males especially after menopause)

Disease Related
- Depression (one of the most common causes of chronic insomnia)
- Anxiety
- Bipolar (manic) depression
- PMS
- ADHD/ADD
- Allergies
- Asthma
- Heart disease and hypertension
- Hyperthyroidism
- Chronic pain
- MS
- Parkinson's disease
- Sleep disorders (restless leg syndrome, narcolepsy, etc.)
- Menopause

- Food allergies
- Fibromyalgia
- Benign prostatic hypertrophy

Lifestyle Habits

- Stress
- Caffeine excess
- Medication side effects (corticosteroids, stimulants, etc.)
- Uncomfortable sleep environment (mattress, noise, temperature, lighting, etc.)
- Alcohol abuse
- Jet lag
- Shift work
- Smoking
- Exercising too late in the evening
- Worrying about sleep
- Excessive napping
- Partner's sleeping habits

Insomnia Treatments

Insomnia that is intermittent or transient may not require treatment since either lasts only a few days at a time. Often removing the irritating factor provides relief — the body naturally adapts within a few days from jet lag, stressful deadlines pass, and so on. However, if fatigue is persistent throughout the day in conjunction with transient insomnia, treatment similar to that recommended for chronic insomnia is definitely warranted.

The crucial first step in any effective treatment plan for intermittent or chronic insomnia is to investigate the cause. This will require a visit to your doctor for a sleep study or further possible testing. In conjunction with this, implement our complete list of sleep tips to create your

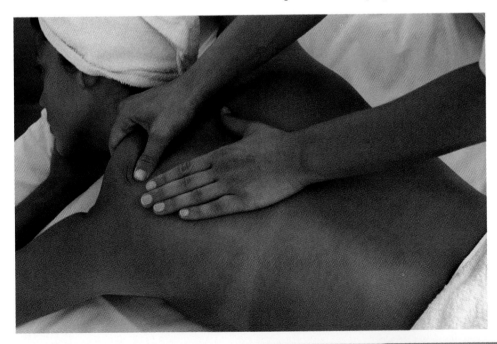

perfect environment and lifestyle habits for sleep. After a few weeks or perhaps sooner, we suggest natural sleep aids to improve the quality and quantity of your sleep if you feel they are required. Both over-the-counter and prescription sleep medications have potential side effects and are not really recommended.

In addition to the sleep remedies listed in this chapter, log on at www.truestar-health.com for natural sleep aids grouped according to their beneficial mode of action, such as sleep disruption due to stress, muscle tension, menopause, and so forth.

Deep breathing, progressive relaxation exercises, yoga, and meditation are excellent for your sleep — just like exercise.

RELAXATION THERAPY: Deep breathing, progressive relaxation exercises, yoga, and meditation are excellent for your sleep — just like exercise. After you exercise, have a hot bath and add Epsom salts to relax your muscles and trigger the sleep response. Soak in water as hot as you can tolerate, with 1 to 2 cups of Epsom salts, for at least 20 minutes. Place a cold towel around your neck if you feel too warm. These techniques reduce or eliminate body tension and anxiety. Relaxation therapy can help your mind to center and calm down, your muscles to relax, and restful sleep to ensue.

MELATONIN: This natural hormone regulates the human biological clock. The body produces less melatonin with advancing age, which may explain why elderly people often have difficulty sleeping and why melatonin supplements improve sleep in the elderly.

Interestingly, double-blind trials have shown melatonin facilitates sleep in young adults without insomnia, but not in young people who suffer from insomnia.

Many doctors suggest taking 0.5 to 3 mg of melatonin $1/2$ to 1 hour before bedtime. However, because melatonin is a potent hormone and the long-term effects are unknown, it should be taken only with the supervision of a doctor.

L-TRYPTOPHAN: This amino acid is converted to serotonin in the body. It is particularly useful for sleep disruption associated with anxiety and depression and for promoting sleep in those who suffer frequent night time waking. L-tryptophan is only available by prescription, whereas a related compound that occurs naturally in the body, 5-hydroxytryptophan (5-HTP), also converted into serotonin, is freely available in health food stores. 5-HTP can help to increase REM sleep, most probably indicating improved sleep quality.

truestarhealth.com

Log on to www.truestarhealth.com for more information on preventive strategies for sleep disorders.

Hypersomnia

At the other end of the scale from insomnia is hypersomnia, or excessive sleepiness. It is an extremely deep or prolonged major sleep period frequently linked with difficulty waking. Although a person with hypersomnia may sleep up to 12 hours a night, naps during the daytime are often needed. If diagnosed as recurrent hypersomnia, it is also called Kleine-Levin syndrome. This sleep disorder typically begins before the age of 25 and its onset is very gradual over time. Hypersomnia may be associated with headaches, fainting, occasional hallucinations, and sleep paralysis.

Causes

Outside of the following medical conditions, the sole cause for hypersomnia is still unknown.

- Major depression (the most common cause of hypersomnia)
- Sleep apnea
- Hypothyroidism
- Anemia
- Chronic viral infections
- Head injuries

Treatment includes good sleep hygiene and stimulants to increase alertness, as well as addressing possible underlying contributing factors if successfully identified.

Restless Legs Syndrome

A condition occurring in millions of people, restless legs syndrome (RLS) causes uncomfortable, overwhelming symptoms in the legs prior to going to sleep, temporarily relieved by movement. The sudden jerking movements to reduce the unpleasant sensations (tension, aching, tingling, itching, or crawling) in the legs and, occasionally, in the arms can lead to insomnia. Symptoms are most common in middle-aged women, pregnant women, and people with severe kidney disease, rheumatoid arthritis, and nerve diseases. Deficiencies of folic acid, iron, and dopamine (a brain chemical involved in controlling movement) have also been linked to RLS.

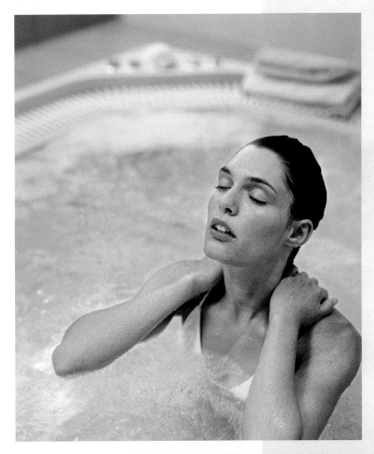

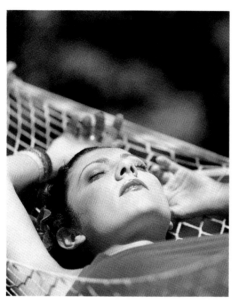

RLS Treatments

Effective treatment for RLS should address the underlying cause (iron or folic aid replacement, kidney support, etc.). In severe cases, symptoms are treated with medications, including those to increase the hormone dopamine, sedatives, or pain medications. Unfortunately, with regular use, these medications lose their effectiveness.

DIETARY THERAPY: Caffeine should be eliminated because it may increase RLS symptoms. A few studies of people with hypoglycemia have reported that 8% have restless legs. In these cases, symptoms improved following a nutritional program designed to regulate blood-sugar levels, similar to the Truestar diet plan (sugar-free, high-protein diet, eating every 3 to 4 hours and sometimes including a night-time snack).

SUPPLEMENTS: Natural supplements offer some relief. Folic acid at a dose of 3 to 5 mg before bed may be particularly useful in RLS, especially if it is familial. Iron citrate can be helpful in cases of iron deficiency diagnosed via blood testing. Gamma aminobutyric acid (GABA), a naturally calming and relaxing supplement, may be beneficial. As a natural alternative to dopamine boosting medications without the risk of side effects, tyrosine (TrueBOOST) can be taken on an empty stomach at a dose of 1000 to 2000 mg daily. Calcium and magnesium supplements assist with normal relaxation and contraction of muscles. Vitamin E may also provide some relief with regular use over at least a 3-month duration. Calcium-magnesium and vitamin E are both found in TrueBASICS, our simple, once daily vitamin pack.

Narcolepsy

Narcolepsy is a disorder characterized by excessive daytime sleepiness and periods of muscle weakness called cataplexy. Cataplexy, the most specific symptom of narcolepsy, is a sudden loss of all muscle tone without loss of consciousness, usually provoked by emotional excitement, such as laughter, anger, or grief. Sleep attacks are short, uncontrollable episodes of sleep during the day.

In the general population, the prevalence of narcolepsy is one in 2,000. Onset is most common between 15 and 25 years, and men are more commonly affected than women. Narcolepsy can be disabling and as severe as other chronic neurological illnesses. It is the second leading cause of daytime drowsiness, surpassed only by sleep apnea. Early diagnosis is important since symptomatic treatment has been proven helpful in this disease. Narcolepsy can result in lack of muscle control, serious problems in one's professional and personal life, low sex drive or impotence, emotional difficulties, and accidents and injury from falling asleep while driving or doing other dangerous tasks.

Symptoms

- Excessive daytime sleepiness
- Cataplexy
- Sleep paralysis and hypnagogic hallucinations
- Disturbed nocturnal sleep (insomnia, tossing and turning, nightmares, restless sleep)
- Sleep attacks

Sleep Paralysis

Sleep paralysis is a lack of normal muscle tone or strength and the inability to move when falling asleep or shortly after waking. Hypnagogic hallucinations are sensations experienced during the transition from sleeping to waking, such as dream-like sequences experienced while awake, often involving visual or auditory hallucinations. Both sleep paralysis and hypnagogic hallucinations are related to the abnormal continuation of rapid eye movement sleep during the transition from sleep to wakefulness.

Causes

The underlying cause of narcolepsy is abnormal REM sleep. A number of researchers believe that a genetic component may be partially responsible for narcolepsy. Studies have shown a 30% concordance rate of narcolepsy in identical twins. First-degree relatives of patients with narcolepsy are 20 to 40 times more likely than the general population to get the disease, yet their overall risk is only 1% to 2%. Autoimmune factors are also believed to play a role in the cause of narcolepsy.

Narcolepsy Treatments

Current treatments of narcolepsy offer symptomatic relief only and do not address the underlying cause of this disease. Cataplexy is treated with antidepressants or other medications to increase serotonin, a hormone important for healthy sleep patterns. Excessive daytime sleepiness is treated with medications to raise the brain chemical dopamine, essential to motivation, alertness and drive. Insomnia is treated with medications to increase sedation or induce sleep like those acting on the naturally calming brain chemical GABA.

SUPPLEMENTS: Although there is not yet a natural supplement that single-handedly treats narcolepsy, a group of supplements may be used in order to support sleep and the nervous system. A good, well-absorbed multivitamin is necessary for general health and well-being. Essential fatty acids

It is the second leading cause of daytime drowsiness, surpassed only by sleep apnea.

(EFA) are necessary for cell membrane protection and for proper functioning of the nervous system. B-complex vitamins are essential for proper brain and nervous system function. Calcium and magnesium are involved in multiple enzymatic and other reactions in the body. Magnesium is a relaxing mineral, which may aid in sleep disorders.

Antioxidants, such as vitamin C, vitamin E, and beta-carotene, prevent free radical damage to cells in the body, including cells in the nervous system. Melatonin has been used in the treatment of narcolepsy and other sleep disorders. Natural supplements of GABA are available in health-food stores or through naturopathic doctors, while supplements of the amino acids tyrosine and 5 HTP can increase the body's natural production of dopamine and serotonin, respectively.

LIFESTYLE: A regular sleep schedule should be maintained as much as possible. Short daytime naps may be refreshing and help alleviate the sleep attacks. Whenever possible, avoid anything that may over-stimulate the emotions and bring on an attack of cataplexy. Reduce stress. Avoiding stimulants such as caffeine and nicotine in the evenings may also be beneficial.

Sleepwalking

Sleepwalking is characterized primarily by walking, but also by removing clothing, going to the washroom, moving items or furniture, or even driving while still seemingly asleep. The individual's eyes are open, talking is typically incomprehensible, and there is no recall of the event upon waking. Episodes can last only a few seconds (just sitting up and lying back down again) to 30 minutes or longer. It most often occurs during the non-REM stages of sleep throughout the night, but can occur in the REM stages closer to the morning. Children aged 6 to 12 are most likely to sleep walk and it does appear to run in families.

Sleep walking can have many causes, including stress, depression, anxiety, epilepsy, or another medical condition. It is associated with a risk of injury because of falls or tripping. There is no treatment specifically for sleep walking. If it does continue, investigation into stress or anxiety should be pursued.

Circadian Rhythm Disruptions

The body is regulated by over 100 built-in clocks that create the circadian rhythm, the 24-hour cycle that paces life's ebb and flow. Each clock follows a unique 24-hour cycle that influences an aspect of the body's function, including sleep, body temperature, hormone levels, heart rate, blood pressure, and even the pain threshold. The body is normally synchronized to a 24-hour cycle of light and dark that we call a day. We are also influenced by the rhythms of the lunar cycle and the change of seasons.

Short daytime naps may be refreshing and help alleviate the sleep attacks.

Although researchers are unclear on how the brain keeps time, they believe that it relies on outside influences to keep a 24-hour schedule. The principal outside influence is daylight. When daylight reaches the eyes, sensory cells in the retina (at the back of the eye) send a message to the brain, registering the presence of light. Other outside influences are sleep, social contact, regular mealtimes, work schedules, and other cues that enable the brain to stay on schedule. The suprachiasmatic nuclei (SCN) areas of the brain act as pacemakers and regulate the circadian rhythm. With age, the brain loses nerve cells in the SCN. This results in changes to the circadian rhythm, such as disrupted sleep and early waking.

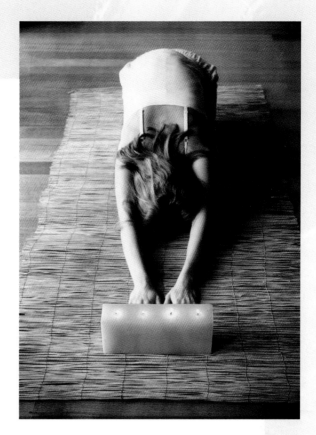

Disruption in the circadian rhythm can lead to a number of disorders, such as delayed sleep phase syndrome (DSPS), advanced sleep phase syndrome (ASPS), jet lag, shift maladaption syndrome (SMS), non-24-hour sleep-wake syndrome, dyschronosis, and age-related sleep maintenance insomnia.

Delayed Sleep Phase Syndrome (DSPS)

DSPS is possibly the most common circadian rhythm disorder and is found mainly in teenagers and young adults, seldom after age 30. DSPS occurs when an individual's body clock is running later than it should be, resulting in sleep-onset and waking times that are very late in relation to the normal sleep-wake cycle. A person with DSPS is unable to fall asleep until well after 1:00 or 2:00 a.m. and has extreme difficulty awakening, usually not rising until late morning or close to noon. People with DSPS sleep the same number of hours as people without circadian rhythm disorders; however, their sleep hours are not synchronized with a normal sleep pattern.

In adolescence, the biological clock normally shifts to a later schedule. Since most teenagers have an active evening social life, study in the evening, or work part-time jobs, they often stay up well past midnight. Going to bed late subsequently results in their being late for school, sleepiness throughout morning classes or even skipping school entirely. The consequences of delayed sleep phase syndrome may be poor grades, family tension, and emotional stress.

The body is regulated by over 100 built-in clocks that create the circadian rhythm, the 24-hour cycle that paces life's ebb and flow.

The consequences of delayed sleep phase syndrome may be poor grades, family tension, and emotional stress.

Advanced Sleep Phase Syndrome (ASPS)

ASPS primarily affects older people. It occurs when an individual's body clock is running earlier than it should be, resulting in early sleep onset and early morning awakening, with an inability to maintain sleep past the predawn hours (e.g., 3:00 to 4:00 a.m.). People with ASPS sleep the same number of hours as people without circadian rhythm disorders; however, their sleep hours are not synchronized with a normal sleep pattern.

Jet Lag

Jet lag is a common traveler's complaint, resulting from travel across multiple time zones. Symptoms of jet lag are daytime sleepiness, sleep disturbance, dizziness, nausea or other digestive symptoms, loss of mental efficiency, weakness, and irritability. It is caused by the desynchronization of the body's circadian rhythm with the new day-night cycle at the traveler's destination and by loss of sleep during the travel itself.

The severity of jet-lag symptoms largely depends on the number of time zones crossed and the direction of travel. Symptoms worsen with the number of time zones crossed. Eastbound travel tends to increase jet lag symptoms, while westbound travel causes less disruption because it is easier to lengthen rather than shorten the circadian rhythm. A flight through six or more time zones may require 4 to 6 days to re-establish a normal sleeping pattern in travelers and to alleviate daytime sleepiness.

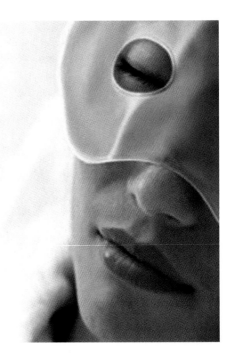

Shift Maladaptation Syndrome (SMS)

SMS is experienced by 40% to 80% of industrial night-shift workers. In a 24-hour period, night-shift workers average 1 to 1½ fewer hours of sleep than day workers. Night workers and rotating shift workers experience sleep deprivation due to a deregulation of the sleep-wake cycle, which disrupts the normal circadian rhythm. In order to conform to a normal sleep-wake pattern, night shift workers usually sleep at night on their days off, thereby reversing any partial adaptation to the night-shift cycle.

After several nights of working and sleeping during the day, abruptly attempting to sleep at normal hours is equivalent to a 6- to 10-hour eastbound flight, resulting in disrupted sleep similar to jet lag. Sleep deprivation and sleep maladaption syndrome are two of the most important factors in decreased performance and increased accident rates associated with night work.

Symptoms of SMS are fatigue, lack of alertness during waking hours, gastrointestinal problems, impaired performance, high accident or near-miss rates, depression, personality changes, and difficult interpersonal relationships. SMS may also lead to more serious health consequences, such as digestive problems and cardiovascular disease. The circadian rhythms of night shift workers should be realigned with the imposed sleep-wake schedule in order to prevent any adverse health effects.

Non-24-Hour Sleep-Wake Syndrome

Most people have a daily circadian rhythm of more than 24 hours (usually between 24.5 and 25.5 hours). Non-24-hour sleep-wake syndrome occurs when individuals are unable to synchronize their circadian rhythm to the 24-hour light-dark cycle we call a day. Although individuals with non-24-hour sleep-wake syndrome continue to function on a 24-hour schedule, their sleep-wake cycle gradually moves later and later each day.

At first, their sleep-wake cycle matches the daily rhythm of life. After a short time, however, the cycle is desynchronized and the individual may have difficulty falling asleep until well into the night. Gradually, the individual becomes unable to sleep at all during the night and experiences extreme daytime sleepiness. Next, the individual is able to sleep in the early part of the night, but wakes early in the morning. Eventually, the sleep-wake cycle moves back into alignment with the normal daily rhythm of life and the individual will sleep well for a short time, until the cycle begins again.

Non-24-hour sleep-wake syndrome occurs principally in blind people, since they have no conscious perception of light. Exposure to light is the primary synchronizer of human circadian rhythms. Researchers have demonstrated that in some blind people, the pathways that transmit light signals to the brain remain intact in the absence of conscious perception of light. These blind people may therefore be able to reset their body clock.

> Sleep deprivation and sleep maladaption syndrome are two of the most important factors in decreased performance and increased accident rates associated with night work.

Dyschronosis

Dyschronosis occurs mainly in children with severe brain injuries. These children sleep in short periods throughout the day and night, resulting in a discontinuous sleep pattern. Dyschronosis is a debilitating sleep disorder that affects both the children and their families. One study reported for children with dyschronosis, nighttime sleep (the longest period of daily sleep) was $2^1/_2$ hours per night on average and that the total daily sleep time was 5 hours, mostly in increments of 15 to 80 minutes scattered throughout the day.

Age-Related Sleep Maintenance Insomnia

Sleeping difficulties tend to increase with age. More than half of all senior citizens (age 65 and over) report regular sleep problems. Seniors often complain about getting less sleep, frequent nighttime waking, early awakening, daytime sleepiness, and frequent napping. In some cases, these sleeping disorders result from an underlying medical condition — arthritis, sleep apnea, and benign prostatic hypertrophy (BPH), or an underlying psychiatric condition, such as depression or anxiety. In most cases, however, the cause of age-related sleep maintenance insomnia is a desynchronization of the sleep-wake cycle with other daily cycles, such as the body temperature cycle, the melatonin cycle, or the light-dark cycle.

Light exposure among seniors, especially those living in nursing homes, is generally much lower than among younger adults. As we age, our body clock tends to run earlier than normal. Advanced sleep phase syndrome (ASPS) may be an underlying cause of age-related sleep maintenance insomnia.

Circadian Rhythm Dysfunction Treatments

With the exception of melatonin, drug treatment has been generally ineffective for the treatment of circadian rhythm disorders.

BRIGHT LIGHT: Bright light treatment, which consists of daily administration of artificial bright light of appropriate intensity, duration, and time of use, has been shown to be very useful in treating a number of circadian rhythm disorders, such as delayed sleep phase syndrome (DSPS), advanced sleep phase syndrome (ASPS), jet lag, problems associated with shift work, non-24-hour sleep-wake syndrome, dyschronosis, and age-related sleep maintenance insomnia. Bright light may be applied to the whole body or, in some cases, applied to the back of the knees.

In the case of DSPS, exposure to bright light, as soon as possible after awakening, has been found to be extremely helpful in resetting the body clock to an earlier time. In the case of ASPS, bright light treatment in the evening, 2 to 4 hours before the scheduled bedtime, will gradually delay sleep onset and, subsequently, delay the awakening time. In the case of SMS, bright light administered close to same

The cause of age-related sleep maintenance insomnia is a desynchronization of the sleep-wake cycle with other daily cycles, such as the body temperature cycle, the melatonin cycle, or the light-dark cycle.

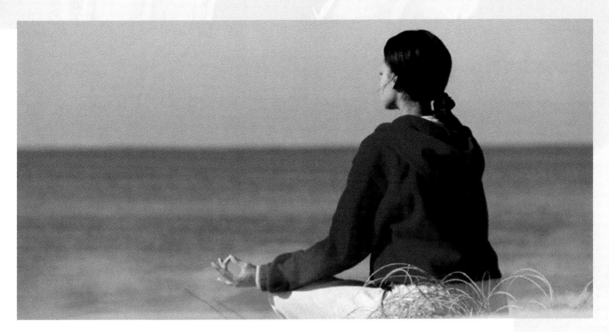

time as the daily temperature minimum, which typically occurs around the mid-point of sleep, could reset the body clock.

In the case of non-24-hour sleep-wake syndrome, bright light treatment administered shortly after awakening may be an effective treatment. Another treatment option is to adhere to a strict 24-hour schedule with social time cues (meals, interpersonal interaction, work schedules) at specific times each day to facilitate resynchronizing the circadian rhythm. In the case of dyschronosis, bright light treatment administered for 45 minutes each morning may be effective. In the case of age-related sleep maintenance insomnia, exposure to bright light in the early evening or late afternoon may lengthen the circadian rhythm of seniors and thereby improve both the quality and duration of their sleep.

LIFESTYLE: The flashing lights of television and video games may reset the circadian rhythm, changing the body's internal clocks. This disruption may result in requiring a longer period to fall asleep, a restless sleep, and waking later during the day. Therefore, television and video games should be avoided, especially by children and adolescents, at least 1 hour before bedtime.

SUPPLEMENTS: Melatonin has been shown to be effective in preventing or reducing jet lag, and occasional short-term use appears to be safe. Melatonin is recommended to adult travelers flying across five or more time zones, particularly in an easterly direction, and especially if they have experienced jet lag on previous journeys. Melatonin may also be used for travelers crossing two to four time zones. Melatonin can be used in the treatment of DSPS, ASPS, and SMS.

Bright light treatment, which consists of daily administration of artificial bright light of appropriate intensity, duration, and time of use, has been shown to be very useful in treating a number of circadian rhythm disorders.

Jet Lag Treatments

- When traveling east up to six time zones ahead of your current time, jet lag symptoms can be significantly reduced by applying bright light during the morning of the day of departure and sometimes for 1 or 2 days before departure.

- When traveling east more than six time zones ahead of your current time, sleep should be delayed and reset at an appropriate time in the new time zone, even if this requires skipping a day, for example, by staying awake for 36 hours.

- When traveling west, stay awake for a few extra hours until the appropriate sleep time of the new time zone. If you have difficulty staying awake, expose yourself to bright light in the evenings upon arrival and perhaps for a few days before your trip. Bright light in the morning should be avoided at the new destination until early morning awakening disappears.

Tips for Diminishing Jet Lag

- Rest well before the flight.

- If your schedule permits, modify your sleep-wake schedule 1 to 2 hours toward the destination's time before the flight.

- Eat lightly before and during the flight.

- Once you have departed, reset your watch and schedule other activities according to the destination time.

- Drink water during the flight and avoid alcoholic beverages.

- If necessary, use caffeinated beverages strategically during the day to mask fatigue. Avoid caffeine within 4 to 6 hours of bedtime, when its effect may make sleep onset more difficult.

- Wear loose, comfortable clothing.

- Schedule outdoor activities during your first few days at the new destination.

- After arrival, adjust to the destination time as soon as possible.

- Limit naps to a single nap of 30 to 40 minutes or less. Go to bed and awaken at the appropriate time for the new time zone.

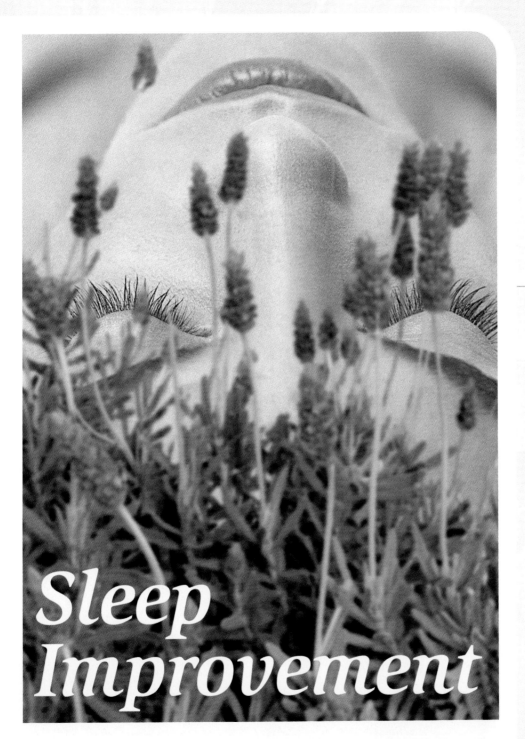

You can use these
sleep improvement
strategies to treat
various sleep
disorders —
and to assist
with weight loss.

Sleep
Improvement

Sleep and Weight Loss

Getting to bed at a decent time has always been said to give you your beauty rest — but now we know it can also help you to achieve a lean body. Good sleep is a key to permanent weight loss. Individuals who are not sleep deprived have an increased capacity to lose weight and keep it off. What is the link between sleep and a healthy body composition? It seems the answer lies in the maintenance of hormonal balance.

Good sleep is a key to permanent weight loss.

Cortisol and Weight Gain

Because of its effect on blood sugar regulation, sleep debt has a harmful impact on carbohydrate metabolism, leaving us at risk of fat gain, especially around the waist.

Sufficient rest and recuperation effectively reduces our stress hormone, cortisol.

When we are sleep deprived, cortisol elevates. Cortisol controls our appetite, often making us feel hungry even when we have eaten enough, raises blood sugar and insulin levels, resulting in increased fat deposition around the abdomen.

To complicate the situation further, high cortisol can negatively affect our sleep patterns, making it difficult to fall or stay asleep when we finally do go to bed. According to a study published in the *Lancet*, sleep deprivation causes an elevation of stress hormone levels in the evening as well as a heightened stress response. This increase in stress hormone also has detrimental effects on other aspects of our endocrine system, such as thyroid gland function, which governs our metabolism.

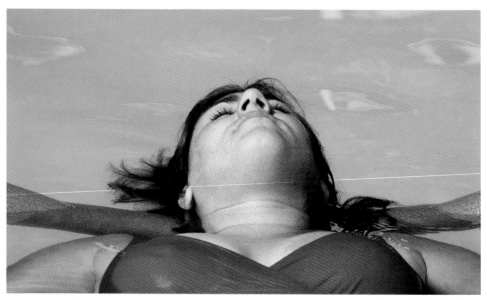

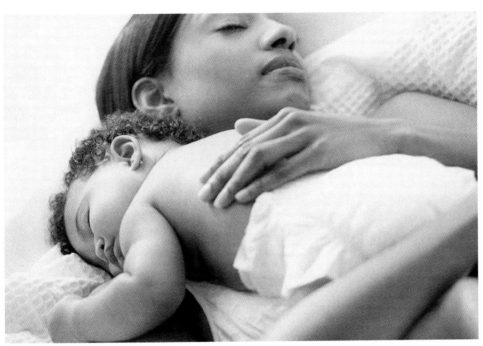

Metabolic Syndrome

Another study recently published in the *International Journal of Obesity* demonstrated a link between the length of time of shift-work and body mass index or waist-to-hip ratio, a marker of abdominal fat. These studies have led to the conclusion that chronic sleep deprivation could predispose to metabolic syndrome and result in an increased risk of cardiovascular disease. The effects are similar to those seen in normal aging. Sleep debt may increase the severity of age-related chronic disorders, such as weight gain and elevated cholesterol or triglyceride levels, linked to metabolic syndrome (insulin resistance), a leading cause of diabetes and heart disease.

Leptin and Weight Gain

Because sleep affects the hormonal balance necessary for effective weight loss, you must watch your sleep habits just as closely as you monitor your exercise and dietary habits. A lack of sleep has an effect on the appetite control hormone leptin. Leptin, produced by our fat cells, acts as a signal to the brain that allows us to determine when we are full or when we should continue eating. Leptin levels naturally increase when we are sleeping and drop when we are sleep deprived. This causes us to feel excessively hungry, and the tendency to overeat is increased. Leptin's appetite-suppressing effect may be the key to weight-loss medications in the future.

Sleep debt has a harmful impact on carbohydrate metabolism, leaving us at risk of fat gain, especially around the waist.

The Truestar Guide to a Good Night's Sleep

If weight loss is one of your goals —
along with your exercise, nutrition, supplements, and positive attitude — you
must get good, restful sleep! Let's move
on to the steps that will allow you the
deep restful sleep your body needs.

If you have trouble falling asleep, if
you awaken too often, if you feel tired in
the morning, if you feel sleepy in the daytime, or if you have a sleep disorder, try
as many of the following techniques as
possible to create the perfect circum-
stances for sleep.

We suggest you try the following
lifestyle habits for at least 2 to 3 weeks
before considering a natural sleep aid if
you feel your sleep has not improved as
much as you would like. Here's our tips
for sleeping well the Truestar way.

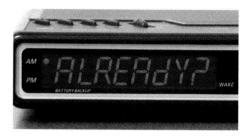

Sleep Hygiene

1. Sleep between 7 and 9 hours per
   night. Oversleeping can be as detrimental as sleep deprivation. If you
   constantly require more than 9 hours
   of sleep per night, see your doctor.
   There are some health conditions,
   such as anemia or hypothyroidism,
   that cause fatigue.
2. Establish regular sleeping hours. Try
   to get up each morning and go to bed
   each evening at the same time.
3. Try to get to bed before 11:00 p.m.,
   optimally, by 10:00 p.m. Our stress
   glands, the adrenals, recharge and
   recover between 11:00 p.m. and 1:00
   a.m, so it is best to be asleep by this
   time.
4. Avoid using loud alarm clocks.
   Waking up suddenly can be a shock to
   your body. If you are regularly getting
   enough sleep, an alarm clock should
   be unnecessary. Sleeping through an
   alarm or needing an alarm daily indi-
   cates you may be sleep deprived. If
   you do use an alarm, you should
   awaken just before it goes off.
5. Sleep in complete darkness. Your
   room should be as dark as possible to
   maintain melatonin balance. You
   should not be able to see your hand in
   front of your face.
6. Do not turn on the light if you go to
   the bathroom during the night.
   Turning on the light, even for just a
   second, shuts down melatonin production and can contribute to sleep
   disruption or insomnia.
7. Turn on the lights or open the blinds
   first thing in the morning. Letting in
   the daylight and the sounds of the

morning imprints the stimulus associated with awakening on the brain. This is the proper way to reset your body clock and ensures that your melatonin levels stay set on 'awake' until the evening.

8. Ensure adequate exposure to sunlight by getting outside during the day. This also helps to imprint a natural day and night cycle on the brain.

9. Try not to nap during the day or early evening — but if you must, keep naps to a maximum of 30 minutes.

10. Do not work past the point of feeling drowsy at night. Go to sleep if the urge comes while watching television, using the computer, or reading.

Diet and Nutrition

1. Avoid bedtime snacks high in sugar or simple carbohydrates and try not to eat in the 2-hour period before going to bed. If you do need to eat something, choose a snack that contains protein, such as a few almonds and half an apple. Protein provides a source of the amino acid tryptophan, which we convert to serotonin and melatonin, hormones important for sleep. The sugars from the fruit may also help the tryptophan reach the brain more easily.

2. Do not drink any fluids 2 hours before going to bed. This will reduce the likelihood of needing to urinate during the night. Men who need to make regular trips to the bathroom at

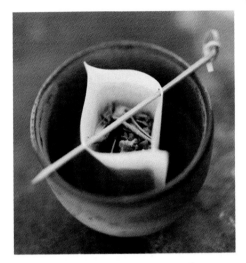

night should see their doctor because it could be an indication of prostate enlargement. TruePROSTATE can offer some relief from this kind of sleep disruption.

3. Avoid caffeine. Not only coffee, tea, and soft drinks may contain caffeine, so do some medications, particularly diet pills. A dose of caffeine usually takes 15 to 30 minutes to take effect and lasts for 4 to 5 hours. In some people, caffeine metabolism may last much longer, making caffeine use in the evening a bad idea. Caffeine may also negatively affect the natural release cycle of the stress hormone cortisol. If this pattern is disrupted, it may keep you awake or cause you to awaken and not be able to fall back to sleep.

4. Avoid alcohol. Although alcohol makes you drowsy, the effect is short-lived. The body metabolizes alcohol as you sleep, resulting in symptoms that can cause sleep interruption. Alcohol may cause

Log on at www.truestarhealth.com to find a selection of meditation and relaxation audios to help you rest, sleep, and rejuvenate each night.

sleep disorders because it seems to affect the brain chemicals that influence sleep. It may also change the amount of time it takes to fall asleep and total sleep time, keeping you from falling into the deeper stages of sleep, where the body does most of its healing. One glass of wine with dinner will most likely not affect your sleep since it takes about 90 minutes to metabolize 1 ounce of alcohol. However, 1 ounce within 2 hours of bedtime or amounts greater than 1 ounce may disrupt your sleep.

5. Avoid smoking and exposure to nicotine. Like caffeine, nicotine can be stimulating and result in increased heart rate, rapid breathing, increased brain activity, and higher levels of stress hormones. This stimulation can make it difficult for most smokers to fall asleep and stay asleep. Smoking can also exacerbate snoring because of irritation on the airway.

6. Avoid foods you may be sensitive to. This is particularly true for dairy and wheat products, as they may affect sleep and serotonin levels. Food sensitivities may result in sleep apnea, snoring, heartburn, nasal and sinus congestion, or gastrointestinal upset.

7. If you are a woman, especially if you are menopausal, eat more estrogen-supporting foods, such as soy, flaxseed, and fennel, to maintain hormonal balance.

Performing relaxing activities in the evening will help you wind down before bed.

Atmosphere and Attitude

1. Keep your bedroom cool — not warmer than 70°F. We naturally feel sleepier when we are cold or are cooling down than when our body temperature is rising.

2. Wear socks to bed. Because they have the poorest circulation, your feet often feel cold before the rest of your body does. Wearing socks to bed reduces the frequency of waking up at night.

3. Meditate in the evening. Performing relaxing activities in the evening will help you wind down before bed.

4. Take a hot bath, shower, or sauna before bed. According to the Mind/Body Medical Institute at Harvard Medical School, we should take a hot bath about 2 hours before bedtime, keeping the water hot for at least 25 minutes to stimulate the drop in body temperature that makes us tired.

5. Do not exercise late in the evening. Exercising less than 3 hours before bedtime may be too stimulating and may impede your ability to fall asleep.

6. Avoid stimulating activities before bed, such as watching television or using the computer. Televisions emit light, which can be disturbing to sleep, and electromagnetic energy, which may increase your risk of cancer.

7. Check your bedroom for electro-magnetic fields (EMFs) produced by electrical outlets, digital alarm clocks, and other electronic devices. If you must

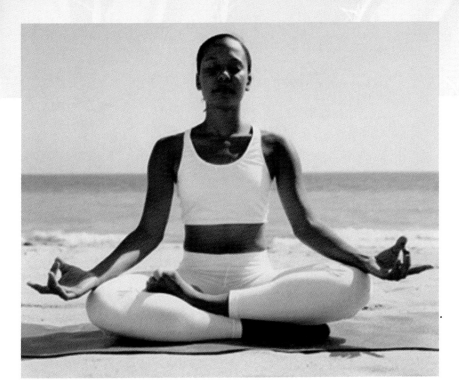

use these, try to keep them as far away from the bed as possible — at least 3 feet away. EMFs can disrupt the pineal gland, which regulates the production of melatonin and serotonin. They may have other negative effects, including increased risk of cancer.

8. Don't work in bed. The bedroom should be a place to relax and enjoy. Use the bedroom only for sleeping and making love.

9. Read something spiritual or listen to calming music. Carefully choose your nighttime music and reading selections — if they are too enticing, stimulating, or suspenseful, you may stay up too late reading.

10. Listen to meditation and relaxation audios. Log on at www.truestar-health.com to find a selection of meditation and relaxation audios to help you rest, sleep, and rejuvenate each night.

Insomnia Aids

1. If you cannot sleep, get out of bed and do something else until you feel the urge to sleep. Lying in bed unable to sleep will leave you feeling frustrated. Staring at the clock will also make your sleepless situation worse, so remove the clock from view.

2. Make a "To Do" list or try writing in a journal if you can't sleep. If you find that you often lie awake in bed with your thoughts racing, get out of bed and write them down. You'll be surprised by how much relief this can provide.

3. Purchase a white noise device or try running a fan if you find that you are easily awakened by sounds.

Exercising less than 3 hours before bedtime may be too stimulating and may impede your ability to fall asleep.

Treatment Strategies

1. Avoid using sleep-aid drugs. Many people who take sleep medications, either over-the-counter or prescription, may experience insufficient amounts of REM sleep, resulting in increased fatigue, moodiness, and irritability. A decrease in life span is associated with the use of sleeping medications and they may become addictive.

2. Check with your pharmacist or primary healthcare provider if you find your sleep habits have changed since starting a new medication. Some medications may affect your ability to fall asleep.

3. Lose weight. Being overweight can increase the risk of snoring or sleep

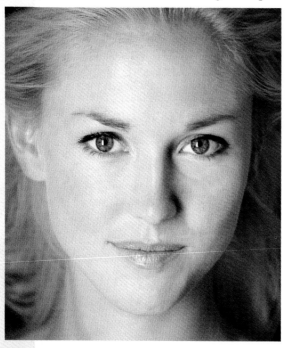

apnea, preventing restful sleep. Luckily the Truestar program is the perfect solution for this!

4. Exercise 3 to 6 hours before bed to maximize the benefits of exercise on sleep. According to the Mind/Body Medical Institute at Harvard Medical School, the body increases deep sleep to compensate for the physical stress exuded on the body during exercise. Exercise also promotes healthy sleep patterns because of its positive effect on body temperature. After exercise, our body gradually cools down and we naturally feel sleepy when we are cooler or cooling down.

5. Exercise your mind. The Harvard Medical School also recommends we exercise our minds. People who are intellectually and mentally stimulated during the day feel an increased need to sleep to maintain their performance. Disengaged, apathetic, and bored people seem to not sleep as well.

6. Have your adrenal glands checked by a healthcare professional. Insomnia may be caused by adrenal stress. This is related to a change in the secretion of cortisol.

7. If you are menopausal or peri-menopausal, have your estrogen, progesterone, and thyroid hormone levels tested. Insomnia may be related to low progesterone levels or changes in thyroid hormone levels. A deficiency of estrogen and progesterone can cause an inability to fall asleep or

truestarhealth.com

Log on at www.truestarhealth.com for more information on natural sleep aids.

stay asleep. Low progesterone levels may also increase anxiety or depression, which often affects healthy sleep habits. These hormones, if discovered to be low, are best replaced with natural hormone creams or herbal preparations, available from your healthcare practitioner. Ensure proper follow-up to measure your hormone levels after using the creams to avoid harmful excess hormones. The hormonal changes that accompany menopause may cause further problems if not properly addressed. Follow the Truestar supplement plan for Women's Health 45+, which may address the cause of your problems.

8. If symptoms persist after using the above remedies and the Truestar supplement plan for women's health, see the herbal remedies for sleep in the following guide to Natural Sleep Aids.

Natural Sleep Aids

Sleep problems affect one-third to one-half of us at some point in our lives, resulting in many of us taking over-the-counter or prescription sleep medications. However, these drugs may cause morning drowsiness or sleep that lacks its natural rejuvenating properties. This is where natural medicines can make a difference.

When taken properly and for the right reasons, natural supplements can be very effective in improving the quality and quantity of your sleep, with few or no side effects. If you have followed our sleep tips for 2 weeks and you have not experienced an improvement, natural sleep aids are your next best option.

Finding the sleep remedy that works for you may be a trial and error process. Luckily, a wide selection of herbal remedies, vitamins, minerals, amino acids, and hormones are available to assist your quest for a good night's rest.

Always remember to use these products in conjunction with the healthy sleep habits we have discussed.

VALERIAN: This herb has been studied for its sedative action and ability to improve sleep quality without the side effects commonly associated with conventional medicines. Valerian mildly sedates the central nervous system and relaxes the smooth muscles of the gastrointestinal

> When taken properly and for the right reasons, natural supplements can be very effective in improving the quality and quantity of your sleep, with few or no side effects.

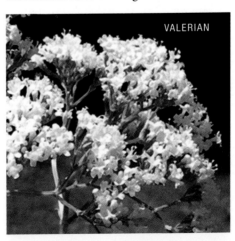
VALERIAN

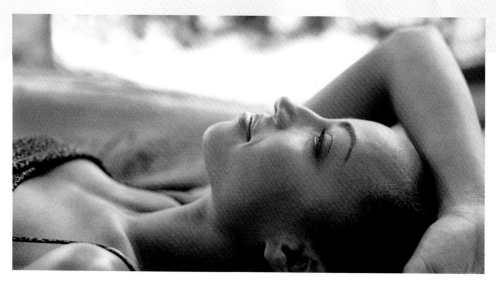

The sleep pattern benefitting from vitamin B-6 supplementation is frequent awakenings, particularly at about 2:00, 4:00, and then 6:00 a.m.

system. Valerian may also be involved in modulating brain activity.

Dose: For treatment of stress, take 200 mg (standardized extract), 3 times per day; for treatment of insomnia, take 200 to 400 mg (standardized extract) at bedtime.

RELORA: This herbal mixture has a calming effect because it blocks the release of stress hormone, excellent for sleep disruptions associated with the typical pattern of waking up between 2:00 to 4:00 a.m. or too early. It is well suited to an individual who is anxious, depressed, stressed, or sleep deprived. It may also assist with menopausal hot flashes.

Dose: 250 mg, 3 times per day away from food.

MELATONIN: Melatonin levels decrease as we age, as well as during times of stress and depression. We recommend a saliva test to determine if you are deficient because melatonin supplements seem only to be useful for insomnia when levels are low.

Dose: 0.5-3 mg at bedtime. Melatonin is not recommended for individuals younger than 40 to 45 years of age. Melatonin deficiency will be more common in the elderly, shift workers, and people with poor sleep hygiene. Higher doses (more than 6 mg per day) should be avoided unless taken under the supervision of a licensed healthcare professional.

5-HTP: A derivative of tryptophan, 5-HTP, is one step closer to becoming serotonin. It may be more effective than tryptophan for sleep loss related to depression, anxiety, and fibromyalgia. 5-HTP helps increase the amount of REM sleep, which is vital to health, and helps decrease the amount of time required to fall asleep, as well as the number of nighttime awakenings.

Dose: 50-200 mg may be taken at dinner or before bed.

VITAMIN B-12: In the methylcobalamin form, this vitamin acts directly on the pineal gland to cause a quicker release of melatonin at night, which resets the sleep-wake cycle. In the early morning hours, it causes melatonin to drop off faster. Overall, vitamin B-12 helps you get to sleep and awaken earlier. B-12 also sensitizes you to morning light, which helps you wake up.

Dose: 3 mg daily to assist with correcting your circadian rhythms

VITAMIN B-6: This vitamin is useful for correcting abnormally high cortisol release throughout the night. The sleep pattern benefitting from vitamin B-6 supplementation is frequent awakenings, particularly at about 2:00, 4:00, and then 6:00 a.m.

Dose: 50-100 mg before bedtime

MAGNESIUM: A natural muscle relaxant, magnesium especially useful if you experience muscle cramps or spasms that keep you awake at night or disrupt your sleep.

Dose: 200-300 mg at bedtime

PHOSPHATIDYLSERINE: This product is ideal for nighttime worrying because it influences the inappropriate release of stress hormones and helps to protect the brain from the harmful effects of cortisol.

Dose: 100 mg at bedtime

ESSENTIAL FATTY ACIDS (DHA): About 60% of brain tissue is made up of fat cells involved in the structure and the transmission of signals across cell membranes. Optimal brain structure and function occurs when the fat cells comprise mostly docosahexaenoic acid (DHA), an omega-3 fatty acid. Serotonin is important for a healthy sleep-wake cycle and mood. Animal experiments have shown that stimulation of certain serotonin

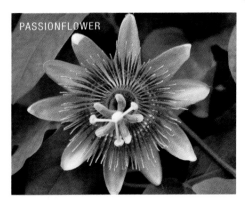

PASSIONFLOWER

receptors leads to a release of DHA from the cellular membrane. It seems that DHA acts as a so-called second messenger within the brain cell, actively participating in the processing and handling of signals related to the serotonin system. Therefore, DHA is important for the regulation of our behavior and sleep. Present findings suggest omega-3 fatty acids, especially DHA, may help in the treatment and prevention of depression, seasonal affective disorder (SAD), and the sleep irregularities accompanying these conditions.

Dose: 1-4 g per day. Fish oils have a natural blood-thinning action and should be used with caution in bleeding disorders or by patients on anticoagulant medications.

PASSIONFLOWER: This is the herb of choice for insomnia because it aids the transition into a restful sleep without any narcotic hangover. It is an antispasmodic, helpful in treating tension and stress. It can also be effective in the treatment of nerve pain, such as neuralgia and shingles. Passionflower extracts have been studied for their potential ability to decrease anxiety and

Passionflower is the herb of choice for insomnia because it aids the transition into a restful sleep without any narcotic hangover.

Log on to www.truestarhealth.com for more information on preventive strategies for sleep disorders.

prolong sleep time. It has also been tested in combination with other sedative and anti-anxiety herbs, such as valerian. Findings suggest that passionflower may enhance the effectiveness of these other treatments.

Dose: For anxiety, 100 mg (standardized extract), twice per day; for insomnia, 200 mg (standardized extract) at bedtime

BLACK COHOSH: This herb is especially useful for sleep disruption related to menopause. Insomnia, night sweats, nervousness, and irritability improve with regular use.

Dose: Crude, dried root, or rhizome: 300-2000 mg per day; solid, dry powdered extract: 250 mg 3 times per day; capsule form: 20-40 mg twice per day. The most thoroughly studied extract provides 1 mg of deoxyactein per 20 mg of extract. Black cohosh should not be used by pregnant or breast-feeding women or by women on HRT. Very large amounts (over several grams daily) of this herb may cause abdominal pain, nausea, headaches, and dizziness.

If you improve your sleep habits, your energy level will remain high and so will your spirits. You will be more successful in your daily activities, and your positive attitude will enhance your health even greater.

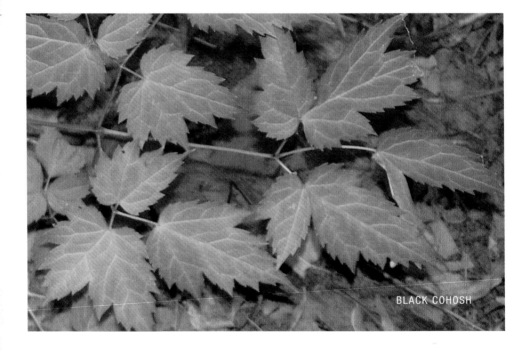

BLACK COHOSH

The Truestar Way

The healthier you become, the better you will sleep, just like the better you sleep, the healthier you will become. It's really a bit of a chicken and egg situation that leaves you wondering which comes first.

If you are tired, you can't exercise properly, you may eat the wrong types of food, be in a foul mood, and likely fail to take your vitamins properly. That's why we've made sleep one of the five principles of the Truestar way to total health and weight loss. If you improve your sleep habits, your energy level will remain high and so will your spirits. You will be more successful in your daily activities, and your positive attitude will enhance your health even greater. That's the Truestar way.

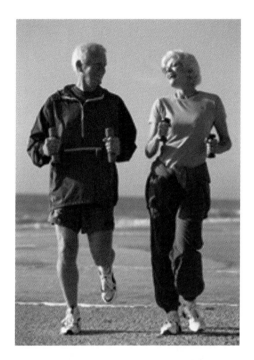

If you improve your sleep habits, your energy level will remain high and so will your spirits.

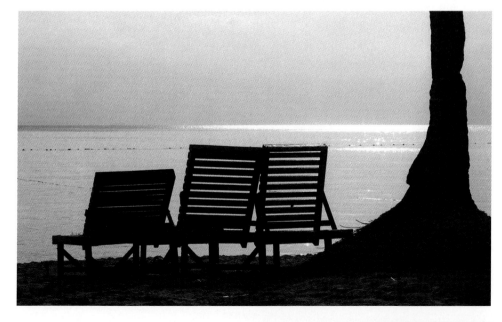

Afterword

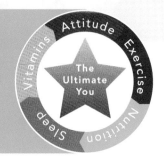

The Truestar Story

Tim Mulcahy
CEO and Founder of Truestar Health Inc.

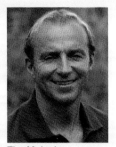

Tim Mulcahy

What started out for me
as a vision of 'selling'
health in a socially
responsible way has
grown into the largest
natural health informa-
tion website in the world
and an expanding
network of health
and fitness centers
throughout North
America.

What started out for me as a vision of 'selling' health in a socially responsible
way has grown into the largest natural health information website in the world
and an expanding network of health and fitness centers throughout North
America.

After the success of the Ontario Energy Savings Corporation public offering,
my interest in selling natural gas dissipated. I felt that I had done the most I
could in terms of personal growth in that industry. My younger brother was
ready to run the sales and day-to-day operations of OESC and has since done a
remarkably good job.

At this juncture in my life, I decided that I would take 2 years off. I'd worked
very hard since the age of 16 and had just crested the proverbial 'hill' at age 40.
Although I had already incorporated the name Truestar Health, I planned to
take some time off to regenerate. I knew that launching Truestar Health was
going to involve a huge commitment and I wanted to be fully prepared, ready for
the exhilaration, challenge, and pace of the ride to my next goal.

After several months of sitting around the house and playing a bit of golf, my
creative energy sagged. I started to become depressed. I had never felt so low,
but, fortunately, I recognized the cause — I was not contributing. I was not
engaged in competing, striving, and creating, all of the activities associated with
being an entrepreneur.

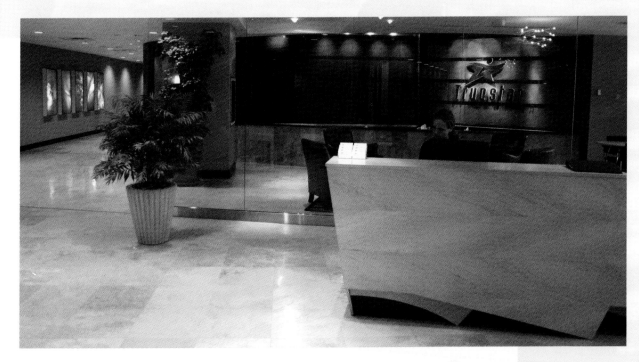

Putting It Together

So, after 7 months of the 2-year hiatus had gone by, I took action. In short order, I rented an office complex and set to work recruiting my Truestar dream team. Our people are definitely our strength. Those who adopt the Truestar way of business thrive early and thrive long.

In this era of the world wide web, I felt that the internet was the perfect platform for Truestar Health. (Truestar was started just after the dot.com bust, or I'm sure another successful IPO would have been imminent right after its formation. Timing is everything; however, learning from what the universe presents and we ourselves create, day by day, is also everything.) Because Truestar was to be web-based, I started off with an IT Project manager. Anthony Whalen, an ex-military officer with specialized project management experience, was Truestar's first employee.

Next came my assistant Alison Greiner, whom I hired for her sales potential in the future, but who soon ended up overseeing our Attitude department for a little over a year. From there, I appointed her regional manager for a district of our soon-to-emerge Truestar for Women Nutrition & Fitness Centers. Alison has since been promoted to be our National Training Manager at Truestar for Women.

I really wanted and needed 'the best' — which led to recruiting Dr Natasha Turner (VP Natural Health), Dr Tudor Bompa (Senior Exercise Consultant) Michael Carrera (VP Exercise), and Dr Joey Shulman (VP Nutrition). Reggie Reyes and Natasha Vani were hired to support Michel's work, Sofia Segounis to support Joey's work.

I really wanted and needed 'the best.'

We set out to sell the best nutrition and fitness program in the industry, backed by a dream team, a website knowledge platform second to none, and a commitment to build something to last — to make that contribution which was missing in my ill-fated 2 years off minus 17 months.

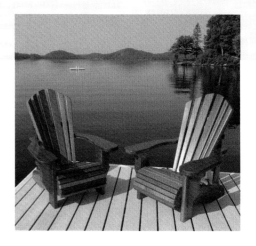

We continue to recruit the best possible personnel for all aspects of Truestar Health. We have added Dr David Schleich (PhD), the former President of the Canadian College of Naturopathic Medicine, as our President. As well, we recruited Terry Nason initally as a marketing director, and later as President of Truestar for Women. Soon thereafter, Rob Crocker joined the team as Chief Financial Officer, Morley Shulman joined to head up our Customer Service operation, and Dr J.J. Dugoua became the director of our multi-disciplinary clinic housed at head office in Toronto. All these individuals believe in our mission and have made a great contribution to the team.

We set out to sell the best nutrition and fitness program in the industry, backed by a dream team, a website knowledge platform second to none, and a commitment to build something to last — to make that contribution which was missing in my ill-fated 2 years off minus 17 months.

Truestar Health is an on-line health and wellness program that gives members a personal program in the 5 key areas of health: Nutrition, Exercise, Vitamins, Attitude, and Sleep. This revolutionary software, created by our IT experts, is on the cutting edge of the health and technology industry. The development of the Truestar website took over 18 months and $15 million dollars.

We proudly launched our 1.2 million-page site in September 2003. Right away, our program brought in members all over the world. We soon had agents representing us on all five continents. The excitement we were generating from appearing on talk shows, being interviewed on radio, and developing television commercials with our strategic partners was unheard of.

As business grew throughout the last quarter of 2003, we identified quickly the one element that was missing from our business methodology — *the personal touch!* People love to work with people. We had a simple, easy to navigate system, but we couldn't reach out and motivate people personally. And so, Truestar for Women was developed, featuring bricks-and-mortar health and fitness centers in communities across the nation. We resolved to take the Truestar way to the people. The business growth of our centers has been nothing short of astounding in the past year.

Truestar for Women was developed, featuring bricks-and-mortar health and fitness centers in communities across the nation. We resolved to take the Truestar way to the people.

Women's Health and Fitness … the Truestar Way

Terry Nason, CFP
President, Truestar for Women

Some people say that I have a visionary, entrepreneurial spirit. I love life and appreciate all the aspects of mine every day. Although I work at it consciously, I have been blessed with a positive attitude, which has always given me a sense of peace, happiness, and adventure. I work to remain always open to the abundant possibilities that unfold every day in our lives. In fact, that's how my relationship with Truestar began.

I have three daughters, ranging in age from 13 to 21, and my commitment to their well-being — to their lifelong health — is total. My life and my family's life changed forever one night a few years ago. My youngest daughter, Nikki, was playing in a hockey tournament. Among the parents who were, like me, cheering on their kids was Tim Mulcahy, who, along with a group of parents, invited me to join them for a drink. That decision to have a social drink with fellow hockey moms and dads changed my life.

The Truestar Vision

At the time, I was a Certified Financial Planner (CFP), responsible for managing assets of individuals and companies, as well as providing consultant services for benefit and business succession. I sized up Tim and thought he would be an excellent client. My firm's extensive services could give him tremendous value. At the same time, I learned later, he was sizing me up as a potential Truestar team member. What began as a plan to recruit Tim as a new client ended by Tim recruiting me. Now, that's selling!

As we talked, my focus shifted away from cultivating a new client to wanting to know more about Tim's vision for his new company, Truestar Health. His passion for this new venture captured my imagination. His synergistic approach to health and wellness, encompassing the principles of nutrition, exercise, vitamins, attitude, and sleep, spoke to my own personal commitment to working out, making conscious nutritional choices, and finding balance in my life. I was intrigued with the simple methodology Tim was explaining. I wondered aloud why no one had thought of this approach before. He shared his plan for delivering personal health programs for everyone via the worldwide web.

Soon after we met, Tim invited me to join Truestar Health as a company spokesperson and Vice-President of Marketing. As the agile Truestar Health Inc. shifted gears, I found myself appointed President of Truestar for Women, a network of fitness and nutrition centers, designed to introduce the five key practices of optimal wellness to women and their families across North America.

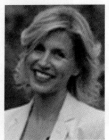

Terry Nason

I work to remain always open to the abundant possibilities that unfold every day in our lives. In fact, that's how my relationship with Truestar began.

What began as a plan to recruit Tim as a new client ended by Tim recruiting me. Now, that's selling!

I enthusiastically embraced the Truestar vision and joined the team. Being proactive on the issue of health and wellness made good sense. I was enthused to be a part of something that would influence so many lives in such a positive way.

Lifelong Health Insurance

At Truestar, I have been able to combine my financial consulting skills and my passion for total health. The financial and the health sectors are both about teaching, leading, and influencing people to invest in themselves, not just for their retirement and financial security, but also for their well-being and their overall health. If you don't have your health, all the money you've made won't be of much value. As Og Mandino has often said, "Who wouldn't give up every last penny for another breath?"

Educating clients to invest financially in themselves and buy insurance to protect their family is important. However, I was only too aware that life insurance only pays out upon the death of the insured — and thus is really death insurance. I wanted to give people *real* life insurance by showing them how to live the Truestar way. This approach to optimal wellness is really about protecting yourself and stacking the cards of life in your favor. Of course, we cannot avoid death — or taxes, for that matter — but we can significantly influence our health and potentially live longer with a better quality of life. What are your health and quality of life worth to you? Priceless!

If you don't have your health, all the money you've made won't be of much value. As Og Mandino has often said, "Who wouldn't give up every last penny for another breath?"

I wanted to give people real life insurance by showing them how to live the Truestar way.

For Women and Families

While developing the extensive health resource at www.truestarhealth.com, we recognized the need to personalize this information if our members were to exploit fully this resource for weight loss and total health. We were inspired to deliver our program to women, one woman at a time. But first, we needed to test the effectiveness of our programs. We decided to conduct a child and family obesity study with 10 families for 6 weeks. Our intention was to teach them the Truestar way and to analyze the effect that this experience had cumulatively on their lives. The Truestar team had one eye on those first 10 families, and the other eye on the thousands of people who would be passing through the doors of our centers and accessing our website.

Attitude

We began by advertising for families interested in participating in our focus group. We had a great response and started to interview. Right from the start, our program manifested its personalized, customized nature. We wanted to ensure that we chose families who were committed to changing their lives. They had to take responsibility for their improvement. We could teach them how, but they had to want to learn how.

Objectives

1. Teach the fundamentals of good nutrition. We wanted our families to learn how to use their personal nutrition

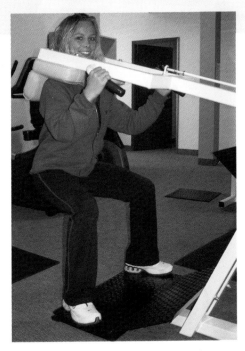

program with confidence and enthusiasm. We even compensated them for the cost of buying nutritious food according to our nutrition plan.

2. Teach how to exercise safely and effectively for weight loss and increased energy. We discussed the science of exercise, including myths and truths. Using the best techniques of interactive learning, we got everyone to step forward and demonstrate the exercises they were learning. We gave them some weights and tubing to enhance their home program. We moved them from idea to action very quickly.

3. Teach the need for taking high-quality vitamin supplements. We supplied each member of the focus group with TrueBasics and TrueLean. This critical element of the program was aimed squarely at educating participants

about the health value of high-quality vitamins.

4. Teach the importance of having a positive attitude. To facilitate this essential dimension of optimal health, we offered motivational input weekly, along with providing everyone with motivational audios and books by leading writers and practitioners, such as Og Mandino, Stephen Covey, Anthony Robbins, and Victor Frankl, among many others.

5. Teach the value of a good night's sleep. Often neglected or simply overlooked in nutritional and exercise protocols, the element of good sleep habits was emphasized repeatedly. We provided each member with tips for getting a good night's sleep.

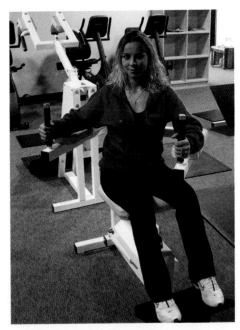

We were inspired to deliver our program to women, one woman at a time.

Right from the start, our program manifested its personalized, customized nature.

Log on to www.truestarhealth.com and click "Find a Center" to locate the Truestar center closest to you.

Procedure

WEIGHT MEASUREMENT

That first night, all family members were weighed, and we calculated their respective body mass index (BMI). The same scales were used to weigh in every time thereafter, and the same qualified person used calipers to measure inches of fat lost. From the get-go, the integrity of the outcome was dependent on ensuring that 'fair testing' practices were being observed at all times.

PROGRAM STRUCTURE

1. We met weekly for 6 weeks at the Truestar head office and fitness center.

2. We started each session with a healthy snack.

3. Every other week (bi-weekly) we conducted a weigh in, calculating BMI and measuring fat.

4. Our experts in nutrition, exercise, vitamins, attitude, and sleep gave presentations and showed members how to navigate the website to find more information.

5. Following a question and answer session, we celebrated success stories.

6. Then each family met with their assigned personal coaches.

Results

We were astonished by the results that our families were experiencing. Not only were they losing lots of weight, but the shift in their attitude and beliefs was remarkable.

The results after a mere 6 weeks were significant:

Total Weight Loss	330.5 lb
Total Inches	220 in

As we came to an end of the 6-week study, we decided to extend the program for five families only for another 4 weeks. The results from this focus group were so positive that we wanted to work with them a little longer to stretch the rubber band and have them experience an even greater level of achievement. We had also committed to a major broadcaster, Platinum TV, that we would participate in a documentary on obesity. For that parallel project, we intended to choose two of

> We were astonished by the results that our families were experiencing. Not only were they losing lots of weight, but the shift in their attitude and beliefs was remarkable.

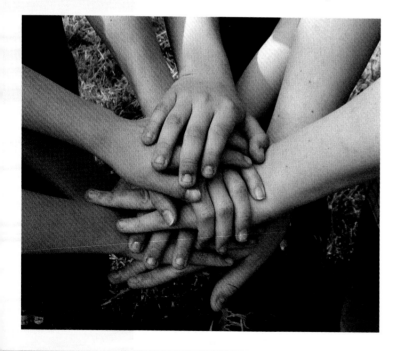

the five families to share their story on this show. Our families were aware of this opportunity and were eager to continue.

We invited the families back to Truestar's Head Office to tape them for the interview that would be included in the documentary. Several of our families were interviewed on local television and radio and in newspapers and newsletters. The media attention demonstrated the public's general interest in real life health stories. "The Truestar Way" was becoming a brand name and Truestar Health was fast becoming a company recognized for being socially responsible to its clients and members.

The final results from the five families were as follows:

Total Weight Loss	366 lb
Total Inches	128 in

Our growing archive of events, testimonials, trainings, seminars and workshops includes those early focus group efforts. Log on at www.truestarhealth.com/press/press.asp for this information and the documentary.

Business Model

Not only were the outcomes of our focus groups wildly successful, the model for Truestar for Women had been soundly established. Optimal health, whether focused on weight loss or not, was going to be predicated on state-of-the-art information, expert advice, constant coaching, counseling and support, and the very best professional standard supplements and vitamins. We had helped these families to transform themselves forever. *Change your life forever!* became our motto. The greatest gift we could have ever given to them was now a proven successful business model for us.

We had the capital, the intellectual resources, the knowledge platform, the health team, and, above all, the desire to bring the most comprehensive, integrated nutrition and fitness program in the industry to the women of the world — the happy intersection of ideas, experience, and action — a winning combination. Just over a year ago, we eagerly started to develop the business model for Truestar for Women. We decided against creating a franchise business, intending to create an income trust.

We wanted to replicate a thousand-fold — a million-fold — what we witnessed with the focus group participants: healthy weight loss, positive attitude, increased energy, better relationships with their loved ones, and a better balance to a stressful life. We wanted to show people how to enjoy their lives to the fullest.

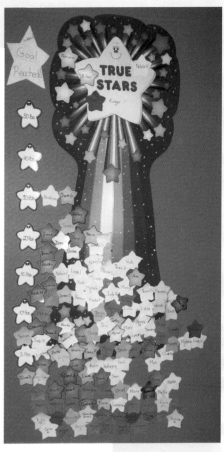

Change your life forever! became our motto.

We wanted to show people how to enjoy their lives to the fullest.

Truestar for Women Health & Fitness Centers

We opened our very first Truestar for Women Health & Fitness Center in Barrie, Ontario. The Truestar Team canvassed the community several days before our official opening and successful booked 120 appointments. We were ecstatic! Our goal was to have 75 to 100 members within our first month, the first of many such targets we have exceeded as our centers sprang up all over Ontario in those heady early months. Our year-end goal was to have 50 Truestar for Women Centers operating — and to keep up this pace annually as we move across the continent.

The success of our centers is based on the understanding that we have the power to make a difference in our society. It begins with knowledge. It ends in the transformation of lives.

Truestar is creating futures, one woman at a time, one family at a time.

Creating Futures

Truestar is creating futures, one woman at a time, one family at a time. Choosing success is as much a matter of attitude, vision, and knowledge as it is energy, focus, and fun. The opportunities for the hundreds of women we are hiring to drive our growth and to serve our members seem to me limitless. The Truestar team is actualizing the dream. We will work diligently everyday to make it come true over and over again for one woman at a time with our commitment, our imagination, and our energy.

Visit us soon at one of our centers or log on at www.truestarhealth.com. Enjoy finding your own Truestar way to total health and weight loss.

Envoi

The Truestar team of experts have enjoyed presenting you with the information in this book, but now is the time to take the next step by converting your knowledge into action. The Truestar Health website at www.truestarhealth.com is also a fantastic tool for developing your own action plan.

You might want to start with these five easy steps, based on Truestar's five principles of health — nutrition, exercise, vitamins, attitude, and sleep.

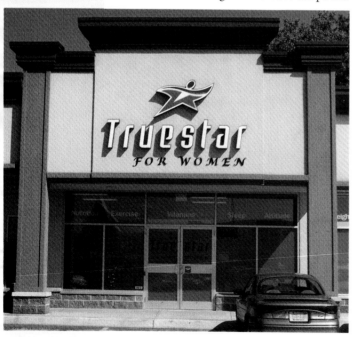

"And in the end, it's not the years in your life that count.
It's the life in your years."   Abraham Lincoln

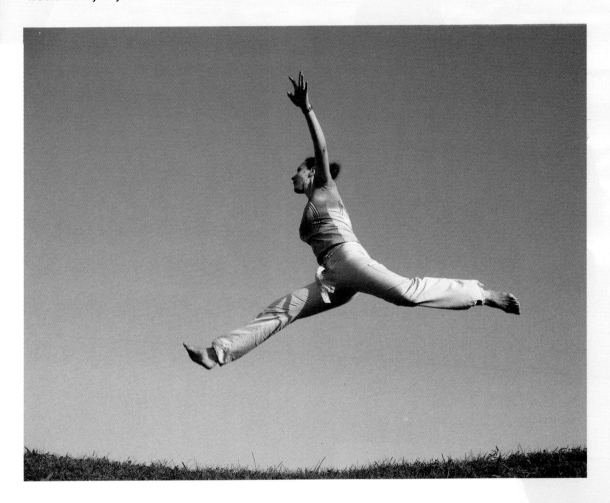

Begin the nutrition program described by Dr Joey Shulman. Try to make one change each day to improve your diet.

Start the exercise program described by Michael Carrera and give it your all. Be sure to consult with your doctor and with the Truestar team to get going.

Determine your vitamin needs as described by Dr Natasha Turner. Begin with TrueBASICS and build from there.

Implement in your daily life some of the ideas for improving your attitude described by Tim Mulcahy. Choose one aspect of your behavior and make a change today.

Improve your sleep habits following the guidelines and tips described by Dr Natasha Turner. Start by going to bed earlier and sleeping 7 to 9 hours each night.

And, as your life begins to change forever, help others by passing the Truestar way on to them.

And, as your life begins to change forever, help others by passing the Truestar way on to them.

The publisher believes the information presented in this book should be available to the public. The nutritional, medical, and health information presented in this book is based on the research, training, and personal experience of the authors, and is true and complete to the best of the authors' knowledge. This book is intended as an informative guide for those wishing to know more about nutrition, exercise, supplements and vitamins, sleep, and attitude. It is intended to complement the advice given by the reader's primary health-care provider such as a medical doctor or a naturopathic doctor. Each person and each situation is unique; thus the authors and the publisher urge the reader to consult with a qualified health-care professional concerning any questions about the appropriateness of the procedures, advice, counsel, or information provided here.

ISBN: 1-894997-14-X

Editor: David J. Schleich
Designers: Larry Harris and Production Plus

Printed and bound in Canada by Tri-Graphic, Ottawa, Ontario.

Co-published by Truestar Health Inc. and Quarry Press Inc.

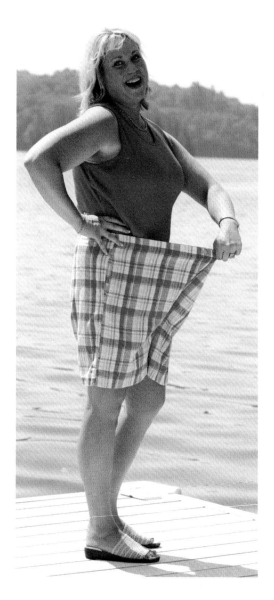

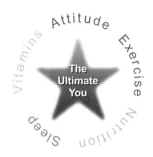

Vitamins · Attitude · Exercise · Nutrition · Sleep

The Ultimate You

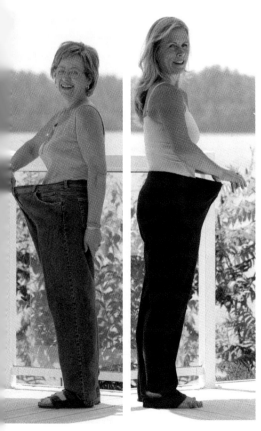

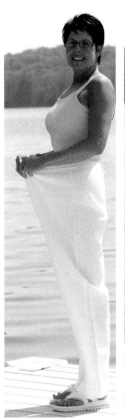

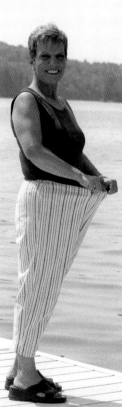